THE
JUMP
START
WORKOUTS

Production of this book is by and for women. Women's rights are human rights.

The typefaces used in this book are:
Twentieth Century Monotype Extra Bold Condensed - book, section, and workout titles
Arial - subheadings on the cover, text on the PAR-Q questionnaire
Arial Narrow - all other text

THE RESEARCH-BASED GUIDE TO BUILDING A BETTER BODY

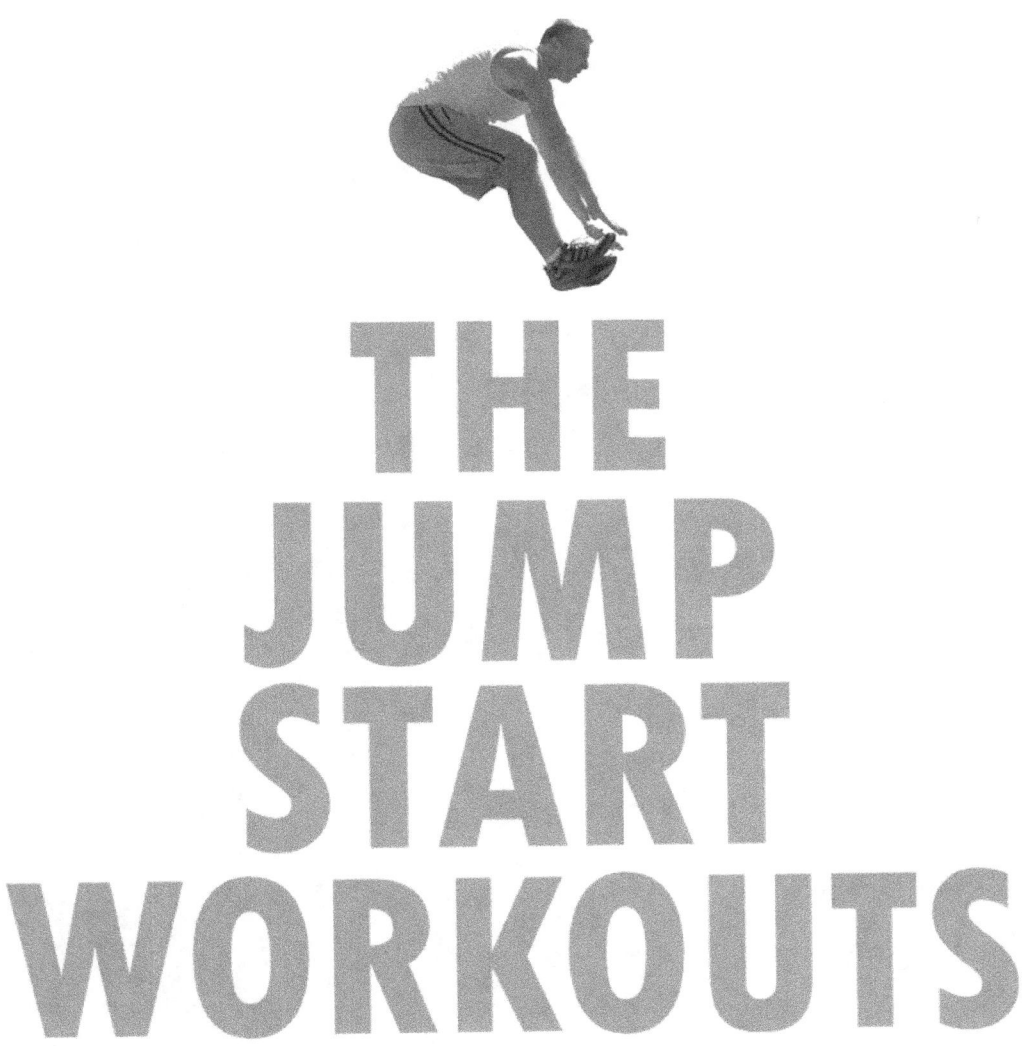

THE
JUMP
START
WORKOUTS

PAUL GROHNE, PT, CSCS

Contents

Section 5 **CONTINUING ON**

Introduction

Your life is your health. This book contains the principles that will improve them both. The better body, vigorous health, and longer life you want and deserve are within your reach. Good workouts are hard, so most people, understandably, avoid them. They prefer to put off the effort of exertion for now and let themselves become too busy to exercise. This neglect ultimately causes more discomfort, in the form of just getting through the day with a body failing from inactivity-related illness, than the workouts would have caused in the first place. Avoid exercise, and comfort eventually vanishes. In the very end, even rest can become unbearable. Working out means putting off comfort now in exchange for more comfort later. Yet the physical discomfort of even the hardest workout is small in comparison to what it creates. Once you've experienced the joy of extending yourself beyond your comfort zone and accomplished a good workout, how hard it is no longer really matters. You will begin to understand that physical fitness and self-discipline go together: the means by which you do the job of working out and the means by which you solve life's problems are one and the same.

The workouts in this book emphasize a most important fitness attribute – strength – but they will also improve your endurance, flexibility, balance, and speed, with exercises built from four basic movements that use your own body weight. Besides one suggested purchase of a pull-up bar (you can buy one for less than $70 and install it in a few minutes, or you can find one at the beach or in the park), these workouts need no equipment. No weights, parking hassles, gym memberships, or traffic jams. Nothing to get in your way. The routines initially require only 20 minutes of your time to start the process of getting you in shape by reprogramming your muscles, your nervous system, and your very mind itself, applying findings from research on exercise science as well as sports psychology to transform ordinary workouts into peak experiences. You'll see how to step up the intensity, without having to lift any weight besides your own body, with movements you've known since early childhood – pushing, lifting with your legs, pulling, and running – and you'll find out how to use these movements to achieve better performance of real-life acts like bending, lifting, reaching, and reacting to a loss of balance while also making real, measurable improvements in your body composition.

The changes you will see from working out happen faster than those resulting from food choices – if someone you know has been working out vigorously for a few months, you notice – and there are plenty of people who work out regularly, eat whatever, and still look good. Of the two, an exerciser who eats whatever would be healthier than a completely sedentary person following a perfect diet. Yet in a world where economic logic compels the mass consumption of low-quality food, you don't want to just eat whatever. Though they accrue more slowly and less visibly, the consequences of food choices add up. The second half of this book will show you a sustainable, filling way of eating that won't feel like deprivation, but will help you lose fat over the long term, and will over time substantially mitigate real health risks. We'll use recipes based on the surprising results of recent research to easily make meals that taste good and digest slowly, yielding a long-burning, high-quality stream of energy. The recipes work together with the workouts in this book to transform you from the inside out.

Beyond recipes and workouts, I want you to understand a little bit of the science behind the choices I'm asking you to make. So, instead of just ordering you to follow my advice, I link each key assertion I make with a citation, using endnotes to list the actual study underlying my advice. As far as I know, this is the only consumer health and fitness book that attempts to support its assertions this carefully. I do this because I think you're smart enough — and, I hope, skeptical enough — to be want the advice you're getting to be supported by specific scientific evidence.

Another reason I spend about half the book describing the science behind its advice is because we live under an ongoing barrage of diet and health information. Interest in effective exercise and healthy eating continues to grow, even as they seem to slip further out of reach than ever. The internet, TV, and radio reporting of health information isn't wrong, but the emphasis, usually on achieving the implausible with the quick and the easy, is misplaced. Segments heralding the latest new study, contradicting last year's study, or thinly disguised infomercials selling supplements whose voice-overs always admit the results depicted "are not typical," can make the simple process of using exercise and food to get in shape seem discouragingly complicated. Some workout routines promote the wrong tool for the job, telling you to do tons of crunches to get washboard abs, for example, or promising superior strength carryover from doing exercises on a stability ball, just as some dietary approaches set you up for future health problems.

Work published in respected peer-reviewed journals like the *Journal of Strength & Conditioning Research*, *Medicine & Science in Sports & Exercise*, the *Journal of Sports Medicine and Physical Fitness*, *Nutrition Journal*, *Obesity*, and others can provide objective, tangible, scientific evidence drawn from systematic assessments of differences in results between one fitness or nutrition approach and another. Research measuring effect, or lack of it, of differing approaches to the problem of improving the human body through food and exercise guide the workouts and recipes in this book. Like they say, science is real.

This book has four sections. First, I organize what I think you would best help you to know about exercise into seven sequential steps, each one building on the other. Second, I put the exercise knowledge into action with four workouts each derived from one of four basic movements and put those workouts into 11 different workout routines encompassing a range of athletic domains. Then, I take the same approach to nutrition, presenting seven sequential steps towards a sustainable way of eating to improve your body composition and health over the long term. And then that's followed by 30 easy-to-make, tried-and-tasted recipes, each with at least one variation, to sustain yourself with a nourishing and rewarding food. One other thing. Write in this book. Make it your own. That will make you an active participant in the process you're about to begin.

Let's get started by using the PAR-Q to make sure you're ready to exercise.

Filling out this Physical Activity Readiness Questionnaire, or PAR-Q, screens you to make sure you're safe for training. It'll clarify if you need to talk to your doctor before starting out. Remember, exercise like any other strenuous physical activity unavoidably carries certain risks. The PAR-Q will reduce but cannot totally eliminate the risk of exercise causing injury, illness, or death. So fill it out thoughtfully, to get your workouts off to the right start.

PAR-Q & YOU

fill this out

PHYSICAL ACTIVITY READINESS QUESTIONNAIRE FOR PEOPLE AGED 15 TO 69

Regular physical activity is fun and healthy, and more people are starting to become more active every day. Being more active is very safe for most people. However, some people should check with their doctor before they start becoming much more physically active. If you are planning to become much more physically active than you are now, start by answering the seven questions in the box below. If you are between the ages of 15 and 69, the PAR-Q will tell you if you should check with your doctor before you start. If you are over 69 years of age, and you are not used to being very active, check with your doctor. Common sense is the best guide when you answer these questions.

PLEASE READ THE QUESTIONS CAREFULLY AND ANSWER EACH ONE HONESTLY:
CHECK YES OR NO.

YES	NO		
☐	☐	1.	Has your doctor ever said that you have a heart condition *and* that you should only do physical activity recommended by a doctor?
☐	☐	2.	Do you feel pain in your chest when you do physical activity?
☐	☐	3.	In the past month, have you had chest pain when you were not doing physical activity?
☐	☐	4.	Do you lose your balance because of dizziness or do you ever lose consciousness?
☐	☐	5.	Do you have a bone or joint problem (for example, back, knee, or hip) that could be made worse by a change in your physical activity?
☐	☐	6.	Is your doctor currently prescribing drugs (for example, water pills) for your blood pressure or heart condition?
☐	☐	7.	Do you know of *any other reason* why you should not do physical activity?

IF YOU ANSWERED YES TO ONE OR MORE QUESTIONS:

Talk to your doctor by phone or in person BEFORE you start becoming much more physically active. Tell your doctor about the PAR-Q and which questions you answered YES. You may be able to do any activity you want — as long as you start slowly and build up gradually. Or, you may need to restrict your activities to those which are safe for you. Talk with your doctor about the kinds of activities you wish to participate in and follow his or her advice. Find out which community programs are safe and helpful for you.

IF YOU ANSWERED NO TO ALL QUESTIONS:

If you answered NO honestly to *all* PAR-Q questions, you can be reasonably sure that you can start becoming much more physically active. Begin slowly and build up gradually, this is the safest and easiest way to go. Take part in a fitness appraisal: this is an excellent way to determine your basic fitness so that you can plan the best way for you to live actively. It is also highly recommended that you have your blood pressure evaluated. If your reading is over 144/94, talk with your doctor before you start becoming much more physically active. Delay becoming much more active if you are not feeling well because of a temporary illness such as a cold or a fever; wait until you feel better. If you are or may be pregnant, talk to your doctor before you start becoming more active.

IF YOUR HEALTH CHANGES SO THAT YOU THEN ANSWER YES TO ANY OF THE ABOVE QUESTIONS:

Tell your fitness or health professional and ask whether you should change your physical activity plan.

INFORMED USE OF THE PAR-Q:

The Canadian Society for Exercise Physiology, Health Canada, and their agents assume no liability for persons who undertake physical activity, and if in doubt after completing this questionnaire, consult your doctor prior to physical activity. I have read, understood, and completed this questionnaire. Any questions I had were answered to my full satisfaction.

Name	Date	Witness
Signature	Signature of parent or guardian (for participants under the age of majority)	

Source: Physical Activity Readiness Questionnaire (PAR-Q) © 2002. Used with permission from the Canadian Society for Exercise Physiology, csep.ca

Section 1

THE SEVEN STEPS OF FITNESS

E ven though I'll be stopping now and then along the way to explain the research behind my advice, what you need to learn from this book about exercise isn't complicated. It's so straightforward that the entirety of the exercise advice in this book can be summed up in a single sentence: Commit yourself to a regular, scheduled program of strength and cardio training to progressively and constructively overload your body. Another way of saying this is to emphasize the importance of the components of good exercise by giving each one of them its own step:

Step 1: Commit Your Time

Step 2: Put Strength First

Step 3: Add Cardio Often

Step 4: Listen to Your Body

Step 5: Endure

Step 6: Intensify

Step 7: Change

As you'll see, each component builds on the one before. Let's start with the first, which lays out how workout success, like most worthwhile things in life, comes to those who take the time, and also shows how to make your workout program accountable to you.

Step 1: Commit Your Time

When you think about it, you get only one body to live in on this earth, so it makes sense to take care of it as best you can. Taking care of yourself is worth your time and energy. With a little effort, a new level of well-being, resilience, and strength is yours to have. Imagine lifting heavier objects, breathing easier, walking more lightly, and being more resistant to injury. These changes happen by doing the exercise in this book. Workouts use exercise like pushing, lifting, pulling, and running to provoke improvement, every time you do them, to make you stronger and any future movement a little easier. The benefits of exercise are well known: healthier muscle,[1] stronger bone,[2] clearer blood vessels,[3] firmer skin,[4] sharper thinking,[5] improved confidence,[6] better aging,[7] and longer life.[8] You've heard this list before, but think about what it means. It reads like a blueprint for happiness. And each element of this happiness blueprint has been shown to relate directly to exercise. The diseases causing us so much unhappiness later in life — killers like heart disease, stroke, and cancer — have their beginning in the health problems of middle age, like high blood pressure, diabetes, and obesity, problems that in turn directly result from inactivity.[9,10] Exercise clears your vessels, elevates your receptivity to insulin (the hormone that brings food energy into cells),[11] and helps you lose fat.[12] Inactivity, really, is poison, and regular exercise is the antidote. And for exercise to work, it needs you to give it some of your time.

All physical activity has value. Working in your garden, doing housework, taking a walk, or simply increasing the time you spend doing your favorite physical activities will improve your physical health. By finding the most strenuous physical activity you enjoy, and doing it more often, you would be following the sage advice of the American Academy of Family Physicians, which shrewdly observes, "The best exercise is an exercise that you will *do*."[13] Yet if good health came from just doing what you already do, the epidemic of fatigue, diabetes, high blood pressure, obesity, and reducible-risk forms of cancer overtaking us wouldn't exist.

So we need something more. As our minds, machines, and communication networks continue to displace the physical labor that in earlier times had kept us healthy, we become tired, fat, weak, and sick. We need to access the benefits of challenging physical work and play during the increasingly short amount of time we have available for exercise. We need to build muscle, burn fat, and safeguard our health with less time out of the day than ever before. Working out can help by giving you the benefits of a day of physical labor within a structured exercise session. In such concentration, exercise can be challenging, but it also gives you the chance to maintain and to improve your body over the course of your entire life.

Assuming you know what exercise to do. So what exercise do you do? Of all the kinds of exercise, the research rather clearly points to two radically different, even opposed, exercise modes that, when pursued systematically, reliably make people fit and healthy: strength and cardiovascular training. Strength exercise, defined as any movement so intense you cannot repeat it more than 20 times before having to rest, builds muscle density, strength, power, and speed. Cardiovascular exercise, "cardio" for short, defined as any movement you can repeat more than 20 times, builds muscle differently, developing stamina and also, as we will see, more efficiently burning fat. They're totally different, even opposed to each other. The best workout program deftly combines both strength and cardio exercise without burning you out.

And where do you work out? A gym can be an ideal place, but not if you're so busy you don't actually go. The workouts in this book require no special equipment so you don't have to actually go to a gym. If you don't go to a gym, don't feel bad. You're not alone. In April 2010, the National Center for Health Statistics reported that fewer than one in four of us engage in a high level of physical activity, and that the overall amount of physical activity people do is decreasing.[14] Other industrialized countries have similarly stories. A 2010 report published by England's Information Centre for Health and Social Care said fewer than 40 percent of British men and 28 percent of British women do any kind of recreational or sport fitness activity three times a week or more.[15] For many of us, our physical activity is limited. We carry only light loads, walking limited distances, and rarely break a sweat. Even those of us who have a current health club membership often don't get there regularly: only on one day out of four (102 out of 365) did members attend their health clubs in 2009, according to the International Health, Racquet, and Sportsclub Association.[16] That suggests that on any given day, do only one in sixteen of us – six percent – actually go to a gym or a health club performing training. That's a problem if the benefits of exercise depend on doing it regularly.

One logical solution to this problem is a a workout that doesn't require the gym. Instead of making you go somewhere to work out, why not a workout that you can do on your own, wherever you are? Instead of having to go someplace to do the exercise, the exercise comes to you. The problems of buying special equipment, of commuting to a health club, and of having to run yet another errand just to get to the gym all go away to be replaced by a more solvable problem, of you motivating yourself to do an exercise session. Hopefully the knowledge you get from this section of the book will help you do that.

Getting more completely informed will also help you work out independently, because you won't necessarily need people working out alongside you or a staff around to answer your questions. That's why it makes sense to learn a little about how exercise works.

So we start with the most basic requirement for exercise, time. There's no way around it: the more time you spend working out, the better your results. Up to certain limits, each additional minute you give to exercise has additional benefit, and these benefits aggregate over months and years of time. The dose-response relationship between exercise and health is pretty clearly established: unless you take it to extremes, the higher the exercise dose, the better your health. The more moments you spend exercising the better you get at it. Your mind and not just your body learns as you go. Over the course of a lifetime, maybe nothing contributes more to fitness than the sheer amount of time you spend on it, yet the good news is if you're new to exercise, you can get discernible results with surprisingly little time.

If physical exertion is new for you, start slow. If you're not used to it, short exercise sessions will initiate changes in your body that will make you stronger by actually reprogramming your nerves and muscles. Doing overly long, intense, or frequent training too soon has long been known to burn out or injure novice exercisers. A well-known study of untrained exercisers published in 1977 in *Medicine & Science in Sports & Exercise* found that participants working out five times a week for 45 minutes obtained only 18 percent more aerobic capacity than those exercising three times a week for 30 minutes, but suffered an injury rate of 54 percent, more than double those with the easier exercise schedule.[18] In this book, novice exercisers start with Workout Zero, a routine of just 20 minutes, three days a week, along with a daily walk. This point, where most magazine article workouts end, is just the beginning.

While safe for novice exercisers, 20 minutes, three days a week won't be enough to keep the positive changes coming. You will need to work up to spending more time exercising if you want to get more improvement. Still, if you are going to put more of your valuable time into exercise, you are entitled to know why. So here's why. The amount of time spent doing exercise has been linked, unambiguously, to muscle gain,[19] fat loss,[20] body composition,[21] and reduced risk of disease in study after study.[22,23,24,25,26,27,28,29] A way researchers compare findings across multiple studies is through a meta-analysis, or "study of studies," which converts the results of different studies into a standardized basis to permit rigorous statistical comparison. One such meta-analysis of some 29 separate studies of women and men doing all sorts of exercise said that the single most important factor for maintaining fat loss over a five-year period was simply the amount of time spent exercising.[30] The workouts in this book will put the odds of success in your favor by having you spend least 45 minutes daily working out.

Slowly but surely increasing your time commitment also readies you for powerful movement that may initially be out of reach. By developing endurance first, then intensity, you follow the well-accepted design of most athletic training programs, which likewise first develop endurance before developing intensity, power, and speed. Thrilling, high-impact movements like the plyometric push-up, the bounding vault jump, or the brief all-out sprint each have their foundation in the

THE DEPARTMENT OF DEBUNKING
QUICKIE WORKOUTS

While better than nothing, workout programs like the Blitz, Curves, or the Eight-Minute Workout do not give you all the exercise your body needs. A Harvard Medical School newsletter warned that such workouts don't, by themselves, prevent disease or weight gain.[31] Think of a quick workout as a gateway, not an end goal, and take heart: each minute you spend exercising makes the longer workouts you need easier to do.

practice of simpler movements done in longer but lower-intensity workouts. Experienced exercisers cycle between longer but lower intensity workouts and more intense sessions of sprints or plyometric strengthening. The principle of laying a foundation of endurance first in order to prepare for challenging movements later underlies the step-by-step exercise approach used throughout this book.

The power of time is indomitable. Nothing, not genetic gift, not age, not money, not access to supplements, compares to it. It may take a while, it may be work, it might be frustrating, but if you put in the time, you will get the results. Other priorities may seem overwhelming, but making time for fitness really makes time for more in your life, not less. A better body, longer life, and greater happiness, the results of long-term athletic endeavor, will come to you with through the time you set aside for honest pursuit of substantial fitness. This time is not lost but sent forward into a better future for you and those who love you. In making time for workouts, you are making yourself better able to care for others by first ensuring you care for yourself. The rest of this book is really nothing more than a logically constructed blueprint for achieving that aim.

So how, exactly, does exercise change you? You'll feel the changes before you see them. During the first four weeks of training, the important changes happen invisibly and on the inside as your nerves undergo a kind of neuromuscular rewiring to achieve faster and better recruitment of muscle fibers even though your muscles will not yet change in size.[32] As training continues, this neural adaptation levels off[33], and if loading demand continues, your body then starts to physically change in response as lean muscle mass increases and fat burns away.[34] Even better, as you persist with exercise, you develop persistence itself. Each workout makes every future workout easier to perform and more likely to happen. In this sense, your success hinges on just simply showing up, an act that over time forges your connection to your best self ever more strongly. Keep at it and the changes will come.

Another way to reinforce your commitment to yourself is by occasionally checking your progress. We'll use girth measurement, a simple but reliable way of assessing your progress that's better than the quicker but potentially misleading bathroom scale. Girth measurement lets you easily and consistently compare the size of your middle (where you store the most fat) and your shoulders, thighs, arms, and legs (where muscle usually predominates). This sidesteps the hassle of complicated body-fat measurement devices, yet gives you tangible, objective feedback so you can see for yourself what exercise routines best help your muscles gradually grow and body fat gradually shrink. There's two easy ways to measure girth.

THE BATHROOM SCALE

It's easy to understand the bathroom scale's appeal: it gives you a number. But it's a number that may mislead you. To get healthier, you want to *add* muscle to your body, not lose it. Since muscle weighs 1.2 times as much as fat, if you're doing your workouts effectively and adding lean muscle, your body weight might not show it. Bathroom scale measurements can be particularly misleading during crash dieting. As you starve, your scale weight plunges as you lose water, and eventually muscle, while your body literally cannibalizes itself for energy. The scale also won't tell you if you're "skinny fat" — average or even below average weight, but with too much fat and too little muscle. Avoid this misery and guide yourself to positive body change, use girth measurement instead.

The first, simplest girth measurement tool already hangs in your closet. As fat tends to be stored towards the middle of your body, your pants size, at least insofar as it reflects the size of your belly circumference, directly relates to your percent body fat.[35] Indeed if you are carrying significantly too much fat, a goal might be to fit comfortably into the next smaller pants size. As your clothes get looser, you will be able to see that your efforts are succeeding.

While a good benchmark, pants or belt size alone doesn't measure change occurring in other areas of your body. Some folks, often men, tend to store excess fat in an apple shape around their middle. Others, often women, store theirs lower on their trunk, in a pear shape along their thighs and upper arms, as well as the middle. To the extent that changes in these areas aren't always reflected in pants or belt size, body girth measurement gives you a way to track your progress more accurately. By periodically checking the circumference of different areas, periodic girth measurements more closely track your body's changing shape. All you need is a tape measure like a soft vinyl tape measure that you can get for five dollars.

Periodic girth measurement will give you the feedback you need to strike the right balance between muscle-building strength work and fat-burning cardio. By giving you a number, it will let you objectively see the result of your individual response to the food intake as well as the exercise of the past month. Whether you use multiple measurements, as on the next page, or the more straightforward pants-size approach, taking girth measurements puts you in control. Taking a few minutes every month to get these numbers might be more cumbersome than hopping on the bathroom scale, but the effort is worth it because among other things it will prove to you that the single factor overriding all others for fitness success is putting in time. Keeping tabs on your body shape might make you think a little more consciously about your choices in exercise and food. The time you invest in doing these measurements will slowly but surely deepen your commitment to continuously improving. You don't have to do it that often, maybe once a month. So for all the reasons, the more accurate information you get, the effect that better information has on shaping next month's food and exercise program, and the reinforcement of your commitment to your program, take a little time at the end of each month to see how you're doing. Here's how. At the end of the month, at the same time each month, perhaps after the last workout of that month before you hop in the shower, grab the vinyl tape measure and do the following measurements. If you're right-handed, it's a little easier to measure your left arm and right leg, if you're left-handed, measure the right arm and left leg:

END-OF-THE-MONTH GIRTH MEASUREMENT: SEE HOW YOU'RE DOING

WHERE	WHAT TO MEASURE
neck	an inch above your collarbone
chest	across the widest part of your chest
waist (belly)	across your navel (belly button), with your belly relaxed
hips	across the middle of your hips and butt
thigh	midway down your thigh, halfway between the hip and knee
calf	across the widest part of your calf
upper arm	across the widest part of your upper arm
forearm	across the widest part of your forearm

Now let's see why the first and most intense of your workouts should, usually, be devoted to training for strength.

Step 2: Put Strength First

Regardless of your age or physical condition, better muscles mean a better body, and the best way to train muscles is to do strength training. There are various ways to train for strength, but for the purposes of this book, we'll define strength training as movements hard enough to do that most people have to stop after roughly 20 repetitions. Endurance training, on the other hand, is what we will call movements that can be sustained for more than 20 repetitions without pause, a category that includes running or cardiovascular exercise.

Many of us shy away from strength training, maybe because it's more intense than relatively milder endurance activities like steady jogging, bicycling, or walking, but strength training has unique benefits that can literally change the shape of your body over time in a way cardiovascular exercise cannot. Strength training even changes the health of your heart in a way that cardio exercise does not, as evidenced by a study of 40 subjects randomized into three groups, of moderate-intensity cardiovascular exercise, high-intensity cardiovascular exercise, and strength exercise, in which only the strength exercisers achieved improved antioxidant status.[36] To make sure you get the benefit of strength training, this book puts it into routines that usually require you to do strength work first, followed by cardiovascular exercise later in the workout or later in the week.

It is hard to overstate the benefit of strength. When you build strength, you become more muscular, toned, and alive with energy. Muscle powers you through the day and makes you injury-resistant by taking load and stress better than any other tissue. Fat weight is dead weight, while muscle weight is live weight. It keeps you youthful as well: one of the most obvious signs of youth is muscle tone. The lateral thigh muscle, for example, of a typical 80-year-old male is significantly smaller (by more than 30 percent) than the same muscle in a 20-year-old male, as measured by a cross-sectional area of key strength-specialized muscle fibers.[37] Matching this measurable decline in size is a decline in the muscle strength between the ages of 20 and 80, also of about 30 percent.[38] While you can't avoid age-related changes entirely, much of this decline may come simply from not exercising; a large-scale survey of 23,000 adults of all ages also showed a decline over a lifetime in frequency of vigorous physical activity. Unsurprisingly, 60-year-olds have been found to engage in vigorous activity much less frequently each week than do 18- to 44-year-olds. How much less frequently? Also by 30 percent or more.[39] Strength work, and the muscle that comes with it, really is a fountain of youth, and we will usually place it first in the workout, so you can give it your best effort.

Another reason muscle-building strength work should be part of your workout is because muscle burns fat so efficiently. Although it weighs 1.2 times more than fat, muscle more than makes up for its increased mass by burning, even at rest, more calories per hour. Each pound of muscle on your body burns about 30 calories a day just resting, while each pound of fat burns only 10.[40] Since lean muscle burns calories, even while resting,[41] adding just a few pounds of lean muscle helps you burn fat away over time. In this way, muscle raises the rate you burn calories, or your metabolic rate, so the more muscle you have, the higher your metabolism.

Given unlimited time, you could experiment with all kinds of ways to build muscle – with abdominal crunches, ball exercises, or smaller movements focusing on just a few muscles at a time. But with over 600 skeletal muscles in your body, it probably makes better sense to focus on exercises that work many muscles simultaneously, especially if you have limited time to work out. Large movements – pushing, lifting, and pulling – can train your body more efficiently because they use more muscles. Instead of doing several exercises for each of your 600 muscles, large movements engage many of them at the same time. By including plenty of such large movements, a good strength-building exercise program is efficient.

In large movements we also encounter the first instance of your body's tendency to adapt specifically to, and only specifically to, whatever you do. This tendency, which we'll encounter again and again in studying exercise, is so ingrained in the human training response that it's called the law of specificity. Always efficient, your body wastes no energy adapting to loads never carried or workouts never done. Instead, you get better with each workout, but only exactly in response to whatever you did in the workout: you get better at what you do, but only at what you do. Exercise physiologists use this law of specificity to design athletic training programs for every aspect of sport performance. Specificity doesn't mean you have to do for your workout whatever it is you're trying to improve at – there are some interesting exceptions we'll encounter later when we look at the effects of higher-intensity training for speed or power – but the truth of specificity, which is that you get better at, and only at, exactly what you do, makes a lot of sense and holds true for a lot of types of training.[42,43,44,45]

This law of specificity suggests that the greatest improvement in real-life physical performance comes from large, real-life movements because they more closely resemble real-life tasks. Real-life movements make you better at handling daily physical tasks, like carrying groceries or walking up a hill. True to the law of specificity, exercises requiring you to push, lift, pull, and move across land will train best train you for the pushing, lifting, pulling, and traveling that make up the majority of life's physical demands.

In one study published in the *Journal of Orthopaedic & Sports Physical Therapy*, 24 healthy adult subjects were divided into two groups. One group did exercises similar to the everyday task of lifting the body with the legs: deep squats with and without barbells. The other group used special exercise equipment, in this case variable resistance machines for knee extension and hip abduction, like the kind you see in gyms. The real-life exercise group obtained better results, not only superior as measured by the amount of weight they could squat three times, which rose by 31 percent (compared to only 13 percent for the specialized equipment group), but also when measured by their vertical jumps, which improved by 10 percent (as opposed to no significant improvement for the special equipment group).[48] The results of this study, and others like it,[49] suggest that for a strength program to be effective, it should include plenty of movements closely related to real life.

Finally, some exercises more than others are better for strengthening your joints and bones. Any exercise requiring you to balance your body against gravity is called "weight-bearing" because it brings load to bear upon your bones and joints. Weight-bearing exercise is good because it stimulates your

THE DEPARTMENT OF DEBUNKING
ABDOMINAL EXERCISE AND SPOT REDUCTION

Concentrating exercise on one area of the body will selectively burn fat away from it, or at least that's how the story goes. This myth is behind workouts involving high numbers of abdominal exercises, but the truth is you lose fat globally and generally, not locally and specifically. Consider a study of the fat content of the forearms of elite tennis players. Because they exercise their dominant playing arm much more than their other arm, if spot reduction actually occurred, their playing arm might be expected to show at least a little fat loss. But magnetic resonance imaging of their forearms showed no difference in fat content between the playing non-playing arms. In fact, the heavily exercised playing arm was actually a little larger because the muscles had grown.[46] In a similar way, doing hundreds of abdominal crunches will not selectively burn fat but cause your abdominal muscles to grow, which will actually make your stomach look *bigger*. Further evidence suggesting the ineffectiveness of abdominal exercises for belly fat reduction appears in a study examining the effects of six weeks of abdominal exercises, which showed no resulting significant loss of abdominal fat, body fat, or body weight, even compared to a control group doing no exercise at all.[47] Since they tend to burn fewer calories than more strenuous alternatives, ab workouts make it harder for you to achieve successful overall fat loss. To the extent that they divert you from more vigorous forms of exercise, abdominal or core workouts can end up perpetuating the problem they were intended to solve.

bone to stay thick and strong. Without at least a modest and regular amount of loading that researchers call minimal essential strain, your bones gradually attenuate over time, becoming thinner and weaker. So scarce is bone-loading activity in sedentary life that by the time most of us reach old age, an ordinary event like accidentally landing hard on your foot after a misstep can fracture it.

Because they're hard, people tend to think of their bones as unchanging, but they actually are a living tissue that changes throughout life. With hormonal and other changes along with less weight-bearing exercise happening as we get older, most of us lose bone mass at the alarming rate of 3 to 9 percent per decade, with women especially at risk after menopause, when hormonal changes and inactivity combine to speed up bone loss further.[50] The resulting bone weakness, called osteoporosis, is a silent but surprisingly widespread problem: often its first symptom is a stress fracture, which more than 25 percent of us experience sometime in our lives,[51] and although prevalence varies with the diagnostic criteria used, about 20 percent of people age 50 or older already have osteoporosis in key bones in their wrists, spine, or hips.[52] Ultimately, this bone loss means that everyday loading events can cause large-bone failures like hip fractures, which remain a leading cause of loss of independence in old age.[53] While a sedentary lifestyle leads to osteoporosis, weight-bearing exercise — introduced gradually to people not used to it — can help. Weight-bearing exercise can stop and even reverse this bone loss, especially in postmenopausal women, who have the highest risk. One study found that postmenopausal women participating in an exercise program that included jumping, running, and strengthening not only increased their bone density but reduced their back pain and lowered their cholesterol as well, while the non-exercisers in the study, even while taking daily calcium and vitamin D supplements, still suffered a 3 percent bone density loss over just two years.[54] The prevalence of osteoporosis and bone's vulnerability to lose density alarmingly fast, even with calcium and vitamin D supplementation, together with the responsiveness of bone to loading, provide additional reasons to give weight-bearing movement a prominent role in your workouts. Weight-bearing movement seems to be especially good for your back: a study from 1983, back when a hospital stay typically included mandatory bed rest, demonstrated that patients on bed rest lost 1 percent of their vertebral bone mass each week.[55] Later research showed that weight-bearing activity (standing, stepping, or balancing) has an even greater effect than muscle contractions (pushing or pulling weight on a pulley) in preserving vertebral bone density.[56] Weight-bearing movements stop bone loss by causing bone-producing cells called osteoblasts to migrate to the site of loading, where they lay down new and stronger bone.[57]

Weight-bearing exercise can help your joints, too. Lacking a direct blood supply, joint cartilage depends on the intermittent compression and decompression of mechanical loading to circulate the nutrient-rich synovial fluid within the joint, which nourishes the cartilage and keeps it metabolically active.[58] Weight-bearing activity is crucial in providing that kind of loading, and by so doing, floods the surface of the joint cartilage surface with synovial fluid.[59] The continued health, strength, and survival of joint cartilage all depend on a variety of loading stresses and strains throughout life.[60] Deprived of compression and decompression, cartilage slowly deteriorates, resulting in the changes that bring about arthritis.[61] The next step presents evidence that running, as a weight-bearing activity, does not seem to promote arthritis, as some people believe, and may even prevent it. I'm not saying that exercise will guarantee you'll never get arthritis, rather exercise should help your muscles, joints, and bones, be as healthy as they can be.

So the workout program in this book will put strength first, with weight-bearing strength exercise to promote strong muscle, bones, and joints, and to closely simulate the motions of real daily life. We turn now to cardiovascular exercise and its own marvelous potential to change your body.

Step 3: Add Cardio Often

Cardiovascular exercise, or "cardio" for short, trains your muscles to use the oxygen delivered by your lungs and heart more efficiently. Whether you walk, jog, or run, cardio activity, when eased into properly, has a snowball effect: each workout makes the next one a little easier, and as their effects accumulate, you'll find yourself not just getting through but really looking forward to your cardio sessions.

Cardiovascular exercise also brings you specific benefits not obtained from strength training, starting with a superior way to burn fat directly, especially for trained exercisers. Provided you do not stop and rest, lower intensity cardio exercise changes your body by burning calories, primarily from fat, as your body first burns through phosphate, then sugar (in the form of glycogen) and other immediately available energy supplies, before switching after as few as three minutes to a steady rate metabolism that efficiently burns fat for fuel.[62]

Because this fat-fueled burn occurs mainly through a metabolic pathway requiring oxygen, lower-intensity cardio exercise is often also called aerobic (from the Greek word for air), which is why we say that fat burns in an aerobic flame. If you want to lose fat, a great way to do it is by doing plenty of cardio (without totally abandoning strength workouts), along with mildly restricting your food intake. This book encourages you to do plenty of cardio, both as structured cardiovascular exercise sessions and through minor changes to your daily habits that significantly ramp up the amount of lighter cardio movement you do throughout your day.

Even better, as you persist with cardio, your aerobic fat-metabolizing capacity improves to enable you to burn fat more quickly and easily. Cardio exercise also strengthens your heart, lungs, and even your blood vessels, with every workout nudging your body towards more efficient oxygen delivery. The mosaic of benefits coming from prolonged cardio training includes greater alertness,[63] lower blood pressure,[64] improved insulin sensitivity,[65] elevated mood,[66] and greater stress tolerance.[67] These changes form a bulwark against the rising tide of obesity,[68] high blood pressure,[69] vascular disease,[70] diabetes,[71] and stress-related health risks[72] brought on by our sedentary life. Over time, regular cardio exercise can prevent and even reverse the severity of many of these conditions.[73,74]

Land-based exercises like walking, jogging, or running make good choices for cardio exercise because they have the associated benefits of weight-bearing activity, that is, stronger bone, stronger joints, and improved performance of real-life movement. They also don't require any equipment, commute, or special arrangements, which maximizes the time you have to get down directly to doing exercise – and burning calories. As we are about to see, the crucial element in any successful fat-loss program is simply burning more calories in exercise than consuming in food, and because they can be sustained for long periods of time, walking, jogging, and running are great ways to do that. A 175-pound person, even just walking at a comfortable 3.5 miles per hour, burns 91 calories per mile.[75]

Running can help you even more, especially if you're pressed for time. The reason running works so well for weight loss is its inherently higher energy cost. Jogging and running not only burn more calories than walking, they even burn more calories than walking per unit of distance. Faster-than-walking forms of locomotion are more metabolically expensive to perform: you could say it's their inefficiency that makes them so efficient. So on a per-mile basis, you'll burn 40 percent more calories, no matter how fast you go, as long as you're going faster than a walk.[76, 77] That's 40 percent more per mile compared to walking, whether jogging slowly or sprinting furiously. Factor in running's faster pace – you cover that same mile faster – and you truly can burn some big numbers of calories. In terms of calories expended per minute, consider the 96, 172, and 293 percent advantage of low, medium, and high-speed running over walking, as the following table shows:

RUNNING: A CALORIE-BURNING JUGGERNAUT

ACTIVITY, MILES PER HOUR	TIME TO FINISH 3 MILES	CALORIES BURNED PER MILE	TOTAL CALORIES BURNED	CALORIES BURNED PER MINUTE
walking, 3.5 mph (17-minute mile)	51 minutes	91	273	**5.4**
slow jogging, 5 mph (12-minute mile)	36 minutes	127	381	**10.6**
jogging, 7 mph (9-minute mile)	27 minutes	127	381	**14.1**
running, 10 mph (6-minute mile)	18 minutes	127	381	**21.2**

It's easy to see how the per-distance calorie cost of jogging or running has the potential to efficiently burn calories, especially for someone with limited time. The advantageously increased calorie-per-mile cost of jogging, to say nothing of running or sprinting, together with the shorter time it takes to traverse the same distance, makes it hard to burn the same amount of energy per day by walking unless you have a lot of time to consistently take very long walks. Then there's its efficiency of access: this form of cardio exercise doesn't require your assembling equipment, traveling, or commuting to a health club. These efficiencies, of per-distance calorie cost, of time, and of access, all make habitual running a potent tool to burn calories, lose fat, and change your body, so much so that it might make sense, even if you think running isn't for you, to think about giving it a try.

Often running is avoided because it's believed it will cause arthritis. While it might be too much to expect running to cure any arthritis you already have, regular running, even over a lifetime, does not seem to cause arthritis and may actually prevent it from worsening. (There are many kinds of arthritis, but in this book, "arthritis" will refer only to the general deterioration of joint cartilage, technically called osteoarthritis, whose symptoms include joint heat, swelling, redness, and pain.) A review of research on running and arthritis shows that even for long distances, running neither causes nor increases hip or knee arthritis, and may even have a protective effect.[78] Evidence also suggests that habitual running relates to no greater incidence of either hip or knee arthritis.[79] Runners may in fact be less likely to develop arthritis than people who never run.[80] A study of 410 runners and 289 non-runners found that vigorous running over many years did not increase musculoskeletal pain, but was in fact associated with much lower disability and mortality rates.[81] In another study of 2,410 people over several decades, low joint-stress activity, like walking, did not increase the risk of arthritis, and high joint-stress activity, like jogging and running, reduced it.[82] A larger Northwestern University study of 5,715 adults found that those *not* getting regular, vigorous exercise developed twice as much arthritis-related limitation as those who did.[83] Still on the fence? Runners live longer, as shown in the Copenhagen City Heart Study, a major 20-year survey of 4,658 Danish men.[84] If research like this is any indication, running should help you maintain and may possibly even improve the health of your joint cartilage without worsening pre-existing arthritis. The slow and gradual walking-to-running activities in this book may help you adapt to running safely.

So far, we've looked at steady-rate cardio exercise done at a single intensity level for a whole session. Higher-intensity cardio training provides additional benefits distinctly different from lower-intensity cardio. At lower intensity, exercising muscles, including the heart muscle, extract most of the available energy in fat and sugar by converting it into glucose and then capturing 95 percent of the glucose energy in a series of chemical reactions dependent on the presence of oxygen. During higher-intensity cardio, muscles revert to a simpler and more primitive metabolism that converts glucose into lactic acid without needing oxygen.[85] (This same anaerobic process occurs in the yeast bakers and brewers use in the fermentation that makes bread and beer.) Even though muscles recycle some of the lactic acid, its buildup ultimately deactivates enzymes, impairs muscle contraction, and causes fatigue and exhaustion.

While that may not sound very beneficial, one result of your body's battle with exhaustion during high-intensity cardio is improved efficiency of the enzyme systems overseeing the lactic acid metabolic pathway — and that translates into improved speed performance.[86] Speed training also burns calories much faster. The calories-burned-per-minute numbers in the far-right column of the table back on page 16 apply only to steady-rate walking, jogging, or running: if you include intervals of higher-speed locomotion, calorie consumption jumps even higher. The distance, hill, interval, and sprint sessions in the workouts in this book will give you the chance to try many kinds of cardio activity, from low-intensity steady-rate aerobic exercise to high-intensity speed training.

Considering the benefits of both steady-rate and high-intensity cardiovascular training, it's no wonder that many exercisers pursue them to the exclusion of other kinds of work. However, the best – that is, the most well-rounded – workout programs combine cardio and its awesome potential to burn calories and improve speed, with equally strenuous strength work, which has the potential to build stronger muscle, joint, and bone, as well as ability in real-life tasks like pushing, lifting, pulling, and balance. Like medicine, strength and cardio comes in doses. The next step will show why.

Step 4: Listen to Your Body

Athletes learn how to tune in to their bodies. They use the stream of information the body supplies during and after movement to adjust loading gently but persistently, forcing themselves to gradually become stronger, faster, and better at their sport. They attend to what their bodies tell them about how much load they can comfortably handle, they learn to apply a little overload beyond what is comfortable, and they learn to do this systematically for workout after workout. This tuning in makes working out joyful.

This ability to listen to your body and incrementally expand your own tolerance for various kinds of load is also what makes physical training work. The effects of these overloads add up, over time, to the entirety of change visible in the well-trained body.[87] The benefits of overloading come from the combination of micro-injuries,[88] enzyme depletion,[89] and temporary exhaustion,[90] small insults that provoke your prodigious capacity to recover and come back even more powerful and resilient. Highly trained power lifters, for example, routinely bench 300 pounds, squat 400 pounds, and deadlift 500 pounds, loads that would break other people's bones. All training improvements and athletic achievements, from the simplest to the most amazing, result from this simple mechanism of controlled, constructive, and incremental overload.[91]

This marvelous capacity to adapt exists in each of us. While it is true some athletes are physically gifted, others are ordinary people who have worked very hard using a disciplined program of gradual and progressive overload to achieve impressive results. No matter what your level of fitness or ambition, you too can learn to listen to your body and use controlled overloads in a safe and constructive way. With training, exercises that might seem completely beyond you now, like plyometric push-ups, jump squats, or wind sprints, become tools you use, whether in full or modified form, to slowly transform yourself.

The same law of specificity that says you tend to only get exactly what you train for also explains why you need to make workouts progressively harder. Your body, ever economical, only makes the minimal necessary adaptations in response to a workout, and will never change further — unless you coax it by taking the exercise further. Most people understandably settle into a workout routine after a while, and fail to keep making incremental improvements. Of course, by doing the same workout, you become able to do it ever more comfortably, and by maintaining your current fitness, you will stay better off than the many who gradually get out of shape over time, but there's always the potential to advance if you're willing to subject yourself to work at full capacity and then some – if you're willing to push it.

Maybe the most important truth of fitness is that meaningful effort is by definition difficult. For that reason those unaccustomed to exercise will find that making an effective level of effort feels uncomfortable. However, if you keep at it, you will find that the sensation of pushing up against your true limits carries a rewardingly sweet feeling of accomplishment. This feeling accompanies very real improvements specific to the kind of limit you have pushed against. A push-up beyond your limit will expand your strength endurance just as an extra quarter mile in your run or swim will extend your aerobic endurance; a slower and heavier squat movement will build your leg muscle strength, and jumping faster or farther will build your core and lower body. To keep going further, you only need to push.

Fortunately, there are so many ways to vary exercise that you will never run out of fresh challenges, even in a workout program consisting of bodyweight exercise. Just learning to work up to and sustain a high level of effort may take some time. Evidence that the capacity for higher-intensity effort develops with training comes from a study of novice weightlifters who, when allowed to select the amount of weight to lift, consistently chose intensities well below the 60 to 75 percent range of their one-repetition maximum. That threshold – 60 to 75 percent – is commonly accepted as the minimum required to stimulate lean muscle growth and strengthening. The subjects selected load intensities of only 42 to 57 percent of their one-repetition maximum. The authors concluded that without instruction, novices select intensities that are too low to get the best results.[92] In this book, of course, we do not use weights, but other ways to pile on intensity.

Obviously, too much overload can be destructive. Exceed your current capacity too quickly, and the weakest link in the chain of nerve, muscle, tendon, and bone will fail, resulting in injury. Training must be controlled. Fortunately, your body comes with a built-in way to measure overload in the form of your ability to distinguish between exertion and pain. While tolerating and enjoying high-effort exercise may be an acquired skill, you already know how to recognize the pain of tissue damage or injury. This is "bad" pain: the sharp, burning, or unexpected pain you get when you hurt your body or aggravate a pre-existing injury. Never push through this kind of pain. Instead, give your instincts credit. Be enthusiastic about gradually pushing yourself harder, and your results will justify your enthusiasm, but stay alert to damaging pain you already instinctively know how to recognize, and heed it as your signal to change or even stop the exercise. To work out safely, modify or stop the exercise if you experience any one of these kinds of pain:

- *Unexpected pain:* Pain in a place where you haven't had it before, or that doesn't make sense to you, is a reasonable signal to modify or stop the exercise.
- *Sudden pain:* If you put too much overload on a weak part of your body, you'll get sudden pain, sharply localized in one area. Never work through this kind of pain.
- *Pain that persists:* Pain that signals you might be injuring yourself continues after the movement stops. If the pain occurs every time you do the movement, lasts after you've stopped the movement, or persists or worsens as you rest, don't repeat the movement. If the pain keeps persisting, you might have an injury, and should get medical attention.
- *Rapidly worsening pain:* If the pain not only persists but worsens minute by minute, even after you have stopped the exercise, seek emergency aid. The more rapidly the pain worsens, the more urgently you likely need help.

As your experience develops, so will your ability to grade your training to provoke change without causing injury. As you continue to work out by listening to your body, you will learn to control the loading effect of work to build, not destroy, and to replace stagnation with a sure sense of purpose, control, and even excitement.

While the advice to push yourself hard but not too hard makes sense, you might want something more specific. How do you know you're pushing hard enough? These two suggestions might bring the advice to push but not break your body into a sharper focus: work up a sweat, but keep any type of increase to about 10 percent a week. These guidelines may help you work out hard enough to get results while keeping you from getting hurt by doing too much too soon.

Let's start with working up a sweat, which is a good sign that you're working out hard enough. About 60 percent of the chemical energy that powers muscle movement is lost as heat,[93] so the onset of perspiration is a reasonably clear indicator that your muscles are moving. Breaking a sweat also correlates with other, less easily assessed indicators of constructive overload, like lactic acid buildup. Even as you get in better shape and break into a sweat less easily, intensity sufficient to provoke improvement still roughly correlates with the onset of perspiration. As your workouts over time make your body more efficient, and you will be able work harder and longer before breaking a sweat, and as you become more conditioned, you'll also find yourself perspiring less during ordinary tasks as your workouts begin to exceed the demands of everyday activity. So think of perspiration during exercise as a signal from your body that you're working out hard enough.

You might also use 10 percent as an approximation of how much to progress training each week. Make any increase – whether in number of repetitions, in intensity, in speed, or in distance – in the neighborhood of 10 percent. Although so far there doesn't seem to be evidence that *not* following this sensible-sounding guideline will get you injured, at least for running distance progression,[94] it has been applied across a wide range of fitness endeavors, from rehabilitation medicine for people with significant impairment to athletes at elite levels of competence. Adding 10 percent more each week should result in slow but exponentially more effective increases that can gradually double your workload in eight weeks and quadruple it in 16. A strength exerciser, for example, might add 10 percent more total repetitions or make a 10 percent increase in his level of effort, while a runner contemplating a month of long-distance training might push herself by adding 10 percent more to her three-mile routine each week, running 10 percent farther. Increasing the same aspect of a workout by 10 percent week after week eventually, of course, leads to absurdity – tacking on a 10 percent weekly distance increase to a three-mile run, for example, would over the course of a year lead to 300-mile runs. In this book, we avoid such overemphasis by regularly shifting focus between three domains of fitness – endurance, strength, and speed – so that you will never find yourself overdeveloping any one area.

So, whatever exercise parameter you focus on, whether it's time spent exercising, number of repetitions, number of sets (a set being a sequence of repetitions without anything but a momentary pause in between them), shortness of rest, total amount of exercise, or intensity of effort, the 10 percent rule gives you a reasonable, concrete, and easy-to-remember way to step up. Therefore, follow the 10 percent rule as a rough guide. Make persistent weekly increases, but by no more than about 10 percent per week, to safely approach your maximum – your personal best – from no matter where you start.

Even though you may initially have to start at a gentler level, you can still use the same 10 percent rule to make progress in your exercise if you happen to have arthritis, joint pain (especially in your shoulders, knees, or back), heart trouble, diabetes, or obesity. These common problems, at least one of which more than half of us have, need not prevent you from training. Of course, use the Physical Activity Readiness Questionnaire (the PAR-Q) on page 3 to see if you need to check with your doctor before beginning a strenuous exercise program. Out of all the common medical problems, it is probably arthritis that might most likely cause you to second-guess your plan to start exercise, even after being cleared by your doctor. On page 13 we looked at how weight-bearing exercise can help joint cartilage heal and may even prevent arthritic changes, and on page 16 we looked at some of the evidence suggesting that jogging does not worsen arthritis. What about general exercise and arthritic pain?

If you have arthritis pain, you may need to go a little slowly, working around whatever arthritis you might already have — although you may not want to push through sharp, persistent, or worsening arthritic pain — but you may be able to participate in more exercise than you might think. In one study, 25 patients with moderate to severe knee arthritis followed a regular exercise program of progressively harder strength training for three months. They experienced less pain as well as improved strength, even on follow-up one year later.[95] The OASIS (Osteoarthritis South Italy Study), a considerably detailed 72-study review, has stated that there is a great deal of evidence suggesting that sedentary people with arthritis should initiate exercise, and that "there is no scientific argument to support halting exercise in case of an osteoarthritis flare-up."[96] Studies like these support the idea that exercise is safe for people with arthritis, at least as long as they don't force themselves to exercise through increasing pain.

By listening to your body, you hone your ability to push yourself without provoking undesirable pain, using this innate recognition in service of lifelong continuous achievement. Through systematic controlled overload (working hard enough to break a sweat and increasing by only roughly 10 percent per week), you now have a blueprint for progress – as long as you're willing to do the work. The next steps show different ways to accomplish this, first by building workload tolerance, or endurance strength, then by further intensifying, and finally by integrating strength and cardio work into a seasonal program of undulating change.

Step 5: Endure

New and experienced exercisers alike usually begin the training cycle with endurance work, which can be pursued through two different modes. Strength endurance involves acquiring the ability to endure a high workload, or volume, of short bouts of heavy resistance against loads such as weights or, as in this book, your body weight, while cardio endurance involves working with or up to sessions of steady-state exertion over the long periods of time. These two modes of endurance training exist somewhat in tension with each other, with strength work building you up and cardio slimming you down. Strength endurance training at sufficient intensity can make you bigger, provoking growth, or hypertrophy, of muscle, tendon, ligament, and even bone; long steady-state cardio sessions result in little if any hypertrophy, and instead will fairly efficiently burn away fat. Despite their distinctly different effects, both these modes of training work together to build up your capacity for physical work and in so doing also build also the self-discipline essential for you to succeed as an exerciser over time. Endurance is work, and your willingness and capacity to do it predicts the extent to which you'll get results from your workouts. Endurance work primes the engine of self-discipline and readies you for tougher workouts in the future. Work begets the capacity to do more and better work, and it is in the commitment of your time, which is most obviously called for in this – the endurance phase – of your fitness program, that you will begin to change. It is impossible after putting in the time it takes to do either type of endurance work not to get something out of it. By teaching you self-discipline, the work you do in the endurance phase of your training reaches beyond just questions of fitness and food to a higher plane of health and happiness. By building up your strength and stamina, endurance work makes all the other workouts possible. The way each mode of endurance training provokes its own specific kind of biologic change is worth a closer look.

With endurance strength training, you start with (or, if you are new to exercise, work up to) a high total amount, or volume, of work by adding sets of repetitions of movements difficult enough to tire you out after less than 20 repetitions. (Remember that a set is a sequence of repetitions without anything but a momentary pause between them.) Much of the research on getting bigger, through increased lean tissue hypertrophy, has traditionally[97] centered on doing a high volume of movements intense enough so that even working as hard as you can, you can't complete more than 10 repetitions: this level of intensity is called the "10 repetition maximum," or 10-rep max. Trying to get by with lower volume has, not surprisingly, been tried. For example, in a recent physical therapy study of 22 untrained older adults, for whom you would expect even modest regular workouts to be of benefit, three months of faithful but low-volume training using only single sets of strength exercise had a modest effect on leg strength — but not enough to have any measurable effect on balance in the women and actually worsened balance in the men by increasing medial-lateral sway.[98] This finding is remarkable because untrained exercisers doing almost any kind of physical training normally show definite improvement while trained exercisers doing the same exercise usually do not. (The ability of untrained exercisers to demonstrate measurable changes in response to pretty much any kind of exercise can confound exercise physiology research by making it harder to identify what works for experienced exercisers. The untrained exerciser effect is so pervasive that it has compelled the adjustment of standards for effect size, so that for a treatment to be deemed effective, the minimum threshold of statistical significance must be set at a higher level for untrained exercisers compared to experienced exercisers.[99]) Going back to the previous study of the 22 untrained adults doing the lower-volume training, the researchers suggested that the exercise program's failure to show performance improvement might have been due to its single-set design using a low volume of required work. High-volume strength training emphasizes sets and repetitions at the 10-rep max intensity,[100] because such training seems to best provoke bodies to get bigger as well as stronger. In a study comparing different protocols for stimulating muscle hypertrophy, the high volume workload (4 sets at 10-rep max intensity) beat out other designs using lower volume and higher intensity (4 sets at a higher intensity of using heavier loads that could only be lifted a maximum of four repetitions, a 4-rep-max) as well as similar volume but lower intensity (2 sets at 25 rep-max).[101] In another study comparing different protocols but equating volume, a 4 sets at 10-rep max design with 90-second rests between sets provoked greater neuroendocrine response, indicating potential for muscle hypertrophy, more than other protocols using higher intensities but longer rests of 3 or 5 minutes between sets.[102] The overall toughness of a heavy workload, at the high but not super-high 10-rep max intensity, with reasonable but not overly long 90-second rests apparently stimulates growth in muscle size by causing a surge of testosterone and growth hormone in men,[103] although the same protocol elicited measurable, if more modest, lean muscle size increases in women also.[104] Such high volume, heavy workload strength training at the requisite 10-rep max intensity has over time become accepted as the optimal workout protocol to increase the size of the muscles used in the exercise.[105,106]

While the 10-rep max can be traditionally and straightforwardly achieved in the gym with weights, many movements in military field training, from which the strength exercises in this book are largely derived, include movements like the pull-up and the single-leg squat that many exercisers will find difficult to do more than 10 times. Other exercises can be done in such a way as to make 10 or even fewer reps nearly impossible – as we will see. In this book, endurance strength work is less about achieving perfect 10-rep max intensity and more about acquiring the toughness and stamina to withstand a high volume of work. If you use proper form, do the full movement, use your own strength, do not "cheat" using momentum, and avoid both within-set resting and overly long (in excess of 90 seconds) between-set resting, just getting through the workout will be hard enough. Most will agree that military field training can get people impressively, even intimidatingly, fit. Army researchers themselves, in fact, faced with the task of training large numbers of people effectively, have compared progressive resistance training using traditional weights with standardized field training strength and cardio work like that used in this book, and have found that field training achieves the same or better improvements on military fitness tests[107] and similar physical performance improvements as derived from traditional weight training.[108]

As you become more experienced doing endurance strength training, you will need to gradually increase the workload to keep getting benefits. To make progress in endurance strength training, we apply the first two of the six methods we will use to make your strength workouts more challenging, by doing 300 and by working to failure. As you become better able to handle the strength exercises in this book, one way to extend endurance in your strength workouts is to count and do 300 total repetitions, regardless of how you divide them between sets. Five sets of 10 repetitions of six different exercises give you 300 total repetitions, as do three sets of 20 repetitions of 15 different exercises. Doing 30 sets of 10 push-ups technically gets you to 300, but it's monotonous: instead of just one exercise, we'll use a variety of them to train a specific movement. Adding roughly 10 percent a week might take you a while, maybe months if you've never exercised before, but by working up tolerance to multiple sets of movement repetitions, you'll be building strength, whether you're a man[109] or a woman,[110] more effectively than you would with an easier workout.

With continued training, you eventually will be able to easily do sets of 10, 15, or even 20 repetitions. So another way to progress further is to stop the counting. Instead of counting to a number that may have become arbitrary, try performing repetitions until you can't do even one more in good form. Good form means holding steady, in control, and without having to cheat by altering the movement. You don't have to know every detail of the exercise: just try to do the movement with your weight centered, in a way that feels right for you. You don't have to work every exercise set to failure, just pick a few sets during the workout during which you try to do as many repetitions as you can. Support in the research for the technique of working until failure includes an Australian study that compared bench press training among basketball and football (soccer) players. It found that the group doing repetitions until failure gained twice as much strength as the group doing a fixed number of repetitions, even though the experimental design ensured that both groups did the same amount of exercise in the same amount of time.[111] Gradually switching from counting out repetitions to simply going until you achieve failure (the momentary inability to carry out the movement in good form) can be a simple way to apply this technique.

What about endurance cardio? The purest form of endurance training, endurance cardio means doing a movement, like taking or running a step forward, again and again countless times, repeatedly and seemingly endlessly, usually in the form of walking, jogging, running, biking, or swimming sessions that emphasize distance.[112] As you propel yourself forward, such steady-state cardio activity enlarges your body's oxygen-carrying capacity, as blood-carrying capillaries and oxygen-processing cellular mitochondria proliferate in the muscles doing the work,[113,114] even as your heart grows stronger and better able to pump blood with a higher stroke volume (the amount of blood pumped per heart contraction).[115] Your aerobic capacity, defined as the maximum amount of oxygen you can consume per unit of body weight per minute of time, also increases.[116] Your mind can be propelled forward as well, into a kind of ecstasy or joy of movement joggers call the "runner's high." Because you do, or can learn to do, such movement seemingly tirelessly and without stopping, and, in time, with a great deal of joy, this highly sustainable form of endurance work, steady-state cardio, is thought to be a primary tool for weight loss. American College of Sports Medicine researchers looking back in 2009 at ten years' worth of evidence for physical activity and its effect on weight loss suggest that strength training – despite its other desirable effects, including impressive caloric peaks – does not enhance weight loss; in fact, it may increase body weight (although this is perhaps because of increased weight from hypertrophied muscle), and so they recommend cardio activity as the primary exercise for individuals seeking long-term weight loss.[117]

Endurance cardio mobilizes and burns fat for fuel,[118] and regular endurance training can substantially enhance your body's capacity to burn fat for fuel during exercise[119] and can lead to substantial weight loss and fat loss.[120] Even better, steady-state cardio training can result in fat loss without lean muscle loss.[121]

Before you surrender to a perhaps understandable urge to turn to cardio-only training and recast yourself as a bicycling god or marathon goddess, consider for a moment further research that seems to contradict the efficacy of pure steady-state cardio for burning fat. Unrelenting cardio work may not optimally reshape you because it by itself does not appear to very effectively build muscle size.[122,123,124] If you're a big person, the prospect of getting smaller without losing muscle may sound just fine to you, but without gaining lean muscle, if you're a pear, years of endurance cardio might only make you a smaller pear, as it did for women who found themselves with increased body fat on their legs after doing only cardio for three months, or a smaller apple, as the men in the same study who ended up after three months of cardio with increased trunk fat.[125] Endurance cardio training did result in lean muscle mass gain in one study – but only in the trunk region,[126] where you might least want it.

Such seemingly contradictory findings might be explained by work investigating strength training's effect on metabolism. In one study, exercisers doing only endurance cardio training lost less fat and also received no metabolic boost, unlike the exercisers who did both endurance and strength training,[127] while exercisers doing both types of training not only achieved superior abdominal fat loss compared to doing endurance cardio only,[128] they also avoided the metabolic slowdown that usually accompanies caloric restriction.[129] Obesity impairs thermogenesis, the ability of stimuli like meals, cold, excitement, and, most crucially, exercise, to raise metabolism, so strength training might be even more important for obese people seeking to improve their body composition. Corroborating such findings are further studies suggesting that steady-state cardio training by itself neither raises metabolism,[130] nor counteracts the body's tendency to slow metabolism in response to decreased energy intake,[131] while a strength training session, by contrast, elevates the exerciser's metabolic rate for 16 hours or longer.[132]

Pure endurance cardio also seems to imperil testosterone, a potent hormone mediating many of the changes we seek from training, from lean muscle mass to red blood cell density. Although testosterone levels are highly individual and not always in lock-step with muscle growth,[133] nor necessarily rigidly predictive of body composition,[134] men have on average about 10 times more testosterone than women (testosterone levels distribute along overlapping bell-shaped curves in both sexes so that some women have more testosterone than some men[135]). Men running at least 40 miles a week had markedly lower testosterone levels than other men, with a similar disparity observed in women runners.[136] Other work notes that chronic endurance-only training suppresses not just testosterone, but adversely affects the entire male reproductive system.[137] There's even concern among cardiologists that ultra-endurance training can damage the heart, with a recent review noting the low mortality and excellent physical function of lifelong vigorous exercisers, but raising concern that extreme endurance events such as marathons, ultramarathons, Ironman Triathlons, and very long-distance bicycle races may lead to calcific or fibrotic injury of heart tissue, particularly in the atria and right ventricle.[138]

In this book, we will avoid the drawbacks of pure cardio by putting strength work first, training to tolerate a heavy-volume strength workload of up to 300 repetitions per workout and judiciously using the technique of working until failure, all while keeping cardio work in the picture – and an alternative track of routines will provide high amounts of cardio for people who want to zero in on weight loss, without completely forgetting about strength training. Before integrating both strength endurance and cardio endurance work into a cyclic workout plan, the next step shows how four other intensification methods from the body-weight strength training arsenal can be used to build strength and power.

Step 6: Intensify

While during the endurance phase strength and cardio work exist in tension between their somewhat opposing aims, during intensity work, they come closer together. Both strength and higher-intensity cardio develop intensity and speed of movement. Neglecting to intensify either strength or cardio means missing out on key adaptations specific to intense movement, which stresses metabolic and enzymatic pathways little used during endurance exercise. Higher-intensity activity calls on a special kind of muscle fiber specialized to perform heavy lifting. These heavy-lifting fibers are thicker, heavier, and help give your body the tone and density associated with being "strong." Finally, strength training is fun. If you've ever played sports, enjoyed an action movie, or solved a difficult carpentry problem, you probably already know something of the thrill of surmounting obstacles through physical force, and something of the sheer joy its proponents call a "fighter's high." This joy of challenge is a reward that comes from pursuing intensification of exercise.

For cardio training, intensification is a straightforward shift in workout emphasis from duration to speed. For strength training, while lifting progressively heavier weight in a health club is certainly logical, we will use other ways to progressively increase intensity without forcing you into a gym. These four ways are: continuous movement, muscle targeting, ballistic loading, and plyometrics. The first two methods can build strength, and the second two build power. As with any other progression, you should apply these intensification methods gradually, using a given method to make your workout maybe 10 percent harder each week. Before we discuss the four methods further, let's take a brief look at intensity training and its physiologic basis in the two types of fiber that make up your skeletal muscles.

Training for intensity takes two forms. The first, strength training, maximizes your capacity to carry heavy load, while the second, power training, maximizes your capacity to move load quickly. Power, expressed as unit of force per unit of time, comes into play during those rare but critical situations in everyday life whenever you catch your balance, adroitly swerve out of the way of an unexpected obstacle, or land from a fall, when your power – your ability to generate intense force quickly – can make the difference between getting hurt and escaping injury.[139] A strong person, like the hulks in strongman competitions on television, can carry the heaviest total weight, but most sports and serious fitness programs also focus on not just the ability to carry weight, but to control it at high speed.

Strength and power movements also call on muscle fibers little used in endurance activities. Why you need to include intense movement in your workout program has to do with the triple nature of your muscle fiber types. Type I – or slow-twitch – fibers, flushed red from iron-containing myoglobin, an oxygen-storing muscle pigment chemically similar to hemoglobin, perform tirelessly, their energy replenished from the oxygen you take with each breath. Walking, jogging, and endurance workouts all train your slow-twitch muscle fibers, along with your entire oxygen-carrying system comprised of the heart, blood vessels, and the capacity to metabolize fat. Yet all endurance workouts target only some of your muscle fibers. Type II – or fast-twitch – fibers, like sleeping giants, need heavy load or powerful movement to be provoked into action. Only exercises recuiring force beyond what slow-twitch fibers can handle on their own can train fast-twitch muscle fibers. Pale, strong, and thick, fast-twitch fibers can generate explosive force, but are only developed by movements intense enough to require such force. A third type of fiber is intermediate, having some characteristics of both. These intermediate fibers are neither as specialized in long-duration oxidative activity as slow-twitch fibers nor powerful as fast-twitch fibers, but they're uniquely trainable, responding to endurance training by gradually changing on a microcellular level to closely resemble slow-twitch fibers and to intensity training by becoming almost indistinguishable from fast-twitch fibers.[140]

So, once you can do 300 repetitions in good form or work until failure, it's time to begin trying some intensification to get your fast-twitch fibers involved. Increasing the weight is the most obvious way to build intensity if you're at a gym, but it may not be the only way. Studies of field-sport athletes (like discus throwers, sprinters, and jumpers) show that the brief but extremely powerful movements required by their sport also train fast-twitch fibers. An often-cited laboratory study of the fiber type composition of the muscles of Swedish athletes demonstrated that while bodybuilder's muscles contained 44 percent fast-twitch muscle fibers, the percentage of fast-twitch fibers for jumping athletes was considerably higher, 63 percent.[141]

Without resorting to equipment, four successively harder intensification methods – continuous movement, muscle targeting, ballistic loading, and plyometrics – vary technique, speed, and length of rest. As we will see, each technique applied in sequence makes the training faster and harder.

Most exercisers instinctively begin applying the first intensification technique, continuous movement, as they become used to a workout routine. To save time, they shorten the rest period between and within some of the sets to shorten and intensify the workout. Shorter rest may be especially effective in promoting muscle growth in men. Frequently cited U.S. Army Research Institute studies have shown that workouts that heighten intensity by shortening rest periods increase blood levels of the two chief muscle-building hormones, growth hormone and testosterone.[142] More recent work has compared 1- and 2.5-minute rest periods and found the shorter 1-minute rest period provoked a greater increase in hormones associated with strength improvement, although the improvements from taking shorter rests appeared to level off after five weeks of training.[143] To apply this continuous movement technique, you shorten the rest period between sets to one minute or less. Then shift your attention to how you do each repetition. During each movement, notice how your body pauses slightly as you switch direction (from going up to going down, for example). Shorten, then gradually eliminate this pause. Ultimately you will be making entire segments of the workout be one continuous, controlled movement from the start of the first repetition to the end of the last. With its short or nonexistent rest periods, the continuous movement workout makes even higher endurance demands than the two previous techniques of doing 300 repetitions and working until failure. This can mean a very hard workout! If you find the continuous movement workout helpful and want to spend 10 weeks progressing towards a workout of 100 percent continuous movement, adding 10 percent per week, go ahead. In general, however, try not to spend too much of your exercise year doing just one kind of workout. Step 7, "Change," will show how to systematically cycle from one technique to another.

A second intensification technique, muscle targeting, concentrates on slow, deliberate movement.[144,145,146,147] During any movement, primary muscles are assisted by secondary muscles and swing, or "momentum," created by the motion. By taking momentum out of the movement and consciously relaxing the secondary muscles, you can target the main muscles doing the movement to make them work harder. To target the primary muscles of a movement, you slow down, focus, and – paradoxically – detach yourself from the motion. This technique can substantially increase the intensity of even ordinary exercises. To use muscle targeting:

- *Slow down.* As you slow down, the motion loses momentum. You have seen momentum at work if you've watched somebody try to lift something that's too heavy by swinging it. Slow down so you have to work harder.

- *Focus.* Attend to your posture and try for perfect form. "Perfect form" means whatever body position best accomplishes the task. You can find this perfect form naturally by positioning yourself in the way that feels just right for doing the movement. As you focus, you will see every movement has two parts: lowering and lifting. Your muscles stretch and lengthen as they give way under the pressure of load, and shorten and contract as they lift. When lowering, breathe in. When lifting, breathe out. Even though the lift usually feels harder, your muscles and tendons experience greater force – and therefore greater opportunity for activation[148] -- as they lower the load. Don't miss out on this opportunity: allow your weight to sink through your muscles during lowering. Make it you alone, not momentum or bad form, powering the movement.

- *Detach.* Once you've mastered the movement, let go of thought. Conscious thinking, especially analysis or self-observation, as we will see later (page 29), actually hurts performance of well-rehearsed movements. As the intellectual part of your brain relaxes its control, the part of your brain in charge of movement can do its job better. Seek detachment. Instead of forcing your body to maximize effort with each repetition, let your will carry you. Your body is no longer the focus of your effort – instead, you are bending your mind.

Suggesting you "bend your mind" might sound a little mystical, but the three-part muscle targeting technique of slowing down, focusing, and detaching can truly create a challenging exercise out of the simplest of movements. As with continuous movement, you don't need to apply this intensification technique to the entire workout to get its benefits.

To understand the third method, picture a linebacker or speeding truck trying to make a sudden turn. It's hard to change directions at high speeds. With ballistic loading, we bring back in force the momentum we had eliminated with the previous muscle targeting technique. The faster you go, the greater your momentum. Ballistic stretching, a perhaps inadvisable practice of stretching by bouncing at the *end* of the range of movement, can tear your tendons and ligaments, but ballistic loading works in the *middle* range, where you still have enough slack to absorb quick shifts in direction. Moving this way turns your own momentum against you, and uses it to load muscle, stress faster-acting muscle fibers,[149] and develop power: your ability to summon the most force in the shortest time.[150]

To use ballistic loading, first consciously relax the nonessential muscles by slowing down, focusing, and detaching in order to target muscles effectively. Then shorten the range of movement so you're neither straightening nor bending all the way: stay close to the middle of your full possible movement range. Staying within a limited range of motion, speed up enough to gain momentum. Before you reach the end of the movement, suddenly change direction. As you speed up, the repetitions begin to resemble oscillations, resulting in a kind of bounce. As you bounce, you should feel a heaviness in the main muscles doing the movement.

Use this technique cautiously at first. Done right, this technique may make your muscles sore. (Actually, any novel exercise can cause soreness, although repeating the exercise may be a cure: one study suggested that as few as two bouts of novel loading movement lessen soreness caused by similar movements for six months afterward.[151]) Perhaps more than any other intensification technique, ballistic loading requires you to pay close attention to form, so you will have to follow the descriptions and pictures that accompany the exercises in this book. As with the other intensification techniques, keep any increases gradual, so that you feel like you're working only about 10 percent harder than however hard you were working the week before. By now, the more intense nature of your strength workouts might require you to take a day off between them, which you can use for a cardio workout.

For the fourth intensification technique, we introduce a new movement: jumping. We'll designate these jumping exercises, some of which also involve pushing off with your hands as well as with your feet, by their proper name, plyometrics. Derived from the Greek prefix *plio-* ("more"), plyometric exercises use high-speed jumping, hopping, and other high-impact movements to further develop strength and speed. A single bout of plyometric training has been shown to nearly double blood testosterone levels.[152] Plyometrics are so effective that they have spread from the athletic field to the health club and even the hospital.[153] While most training follows the specificity law, giving you only the improvements that you train for, some evidence suggests plyometrics may confer additional benefits beyond just better performance of plyometric exercise itself. Distance runners undergoing six weeks of plyometric training, for example, improved not only plyometric performance, but also their running economy.[154] (Like gas mileage, running economy is a measure of how much distance is covered per unit of fuel.) Plyometric exercise also enhanced one-repetition maximum squat performance under a heavy weight.[155] That plyometric work seems to positively influence such seemingly unrelated aspects of fitness – maximal strength, endurance efficiency, and androgenic hormone levels – suggests that its contribution to human movement capability may be very fundamental.

High in speed and explosive in intensity, plyometrics can become part of your workouts if you use common sense. The workout instructions will show you how to modify the movement to make it easy enough for you to do without hurting yourself. If you have a bone, joint, or balance problem, or if you're just not used to intense exercise, skip plyometric movement altogether until you've built up a base of strength and conditioning first. Think of plyometric movement as a possibility, not something you have to do. Before attempting plyometrics, you should be able to do three full-range single-leg squats, five clap pushups in good form, and a 100-yard sprint at your perceived maximum, tasks you will eventually be able to perform if you persist with training. (These plyometric prerequisites appear later alongside the plyometric exercises introduced in Workout 1 on page 38 and again in Workout 3 on page 45.) As with the other intensification techniques, you need not do a 100-percent-plyometric workout to get its benefit; if you wish to devote more than 10 to 20 percent of your workout to plyometric intensification, do so in 10 percent increments (for example, 40 percent of the workout on plyometrics the first week, 50 percent the second, and so on for four weeks with the final week being mostly plyometrics). Finally, schedule a day of recovery or cardio between plyometric days.

We have looked at four ways to intensify: continuous movement, muscle targeting, ballistic loading, and plyometrics, all of them physical. What about intensifying the mental component of exercise? We saw how focusing yet relaxing helps you target your muscles. Let's look more closely at the mind-body connection in exercise and what research says about the brain, which really is the one organ most determinant of your success with training.

High-achieving exercisers and athletes have the ability to work out intensely, over and over, without experiencing it as drudgery. Whether athletes, artists, or executives, peak performers enjoy their work. While working at their highest level they achieve a sense of effortlessness, an absence of fear, and a profound sense of control. People who enjoy exercise the most and perform more often at their best achieve this state of awareness, which athletes call "being in the zone." The reduced brainwave activity (as measured by electroencephalography) during elite athletes' performance of difficult physical tasks is ascribed to their success in shutting out distractions and narrowing their focus.[156] Can you learn to think like they do, enjoying your exercise more, even as you perform it better, by sharpening your mind as well as your body?

After sufficient practice, thinking too much about your performance can hamper the natural efficiencies your active brain manages *without* the conscious interference of your thinking brain. For example, Mike Stanley was playing catcher for the Texas Rangers when he began to pay attention to his throwing percentage (the percentage of base runners a catcher throws out). His performance deteriorated – he threw rainbows to second and third base and short lobs back to the pitcher. After being coached simply not to think so much about his throw, he began to throw with a much surer arm. "My arm is the same as before," Stanley reflected. "I'm just not afraid to let it go anymore."[157] Think of peak movement performance as letting your heart and soul – not just your thinking brain – guide you. You'll enjoy the exercise more as you learn an easier way of driving the movement: you just let it happen. Getting in the flow means not a loss of focus, but a shift of focus. It means attending to the movement, but by shifting your attention outside of yourself. Giving some intellectual rigor to the dreamy idea of letting your soul and not your meddlesome consciousness guide movement is the constraint theory of motor learning, which explains why performers who focus externally instead of internally do better. Each of us have unique attributes that impact movement, like the length of the lower leg, or the ratio between ankle joint stiffness and the length of the foot, that interact with hundreds of other individual physical constraints to result in a number of possible movements from which one way is the easiest, most efficient, and least metabolically costly way to get the job done. Our moving brain marvelously and innately finds that way, and perhaps finds it more quickly with less interference from the conscious mind. That's why basketball students, in an eloquent example from a recent study summing up some 15 years of motor learning research,[158] instructed to listen for an even and audible sound of the basketball striking the floor (an external focus), achieved better performance than those coached to push the ball down with even movements of wrist and hand (an internal focus). The 84 sprinters in the same study likewise enjoyed improved performance when instructed to externally focus their attention.

With the addition of continuous movement, muscle targeting, ballistic loading, and plyometrics, we now have four successively harder ways to intensify your training without having to use a gym. You also know that some of the fire that burns within star performers isn't completely mysterious, but can to some extent be developed by practice.

Step 7: Change

By now, our workout equation has a lot of variables: two modes of exercise (strength and cardio), six successive intensification techniques (doing 300, working until failure, continuous movement, muscle targeting, ballistic loading, and plyometrics), three levels of intensity (endurance, strength, and speed), and five types of movement (pushing, lifting, jumping, pulling, and running). So how do you put these all together? How do you integrate all these variables into a simple routine of activity, balance the opposing effects of strength and cardio, get stronger without getting slower and faster without getting weaker, and stay interested in exercise without burning out? Athletes achieve these objectives by using a technique called periodization to systematically change workout emphasis over time.[159]

Your workouts should, as the routines in this book do, gradually shift from building endurance to intensifying and finally to speed and performance. The workout routines presented later on take the guesswork out of what workout to do when, but this last step, "Change," will show you how to manipulate the frequency, intensity, and focus of cardio and strength workouts yourself over days, weeks, and months, shifting first from foundation-building endurance to intensification and strength, and then to speed-training and power in order to give you undistracted focus on each fitness domain and also to keep your exercise program fresh and ever evolving for the rest of your life. This section of the book will complete the knowledge you need to take charge of your exercise program by showing you how periodization works. The routines ahead do the periodization for you, but before you do them, read on to understand a little bit about how periodization can maximize exercise performance.

First, does periodization work? Yes. Research suggests that periodized workout programs get better results than non-periodized workouts, for both cardio[160] and strength training.[161] Among the evidence in favor of periodization is a review finding that non-periodized training (sometimes called "mixed training") lacks peak performance experiences, provides insufficient or conflicting training stimuli, and can burn exercisers out. The review suggests focusing on one target for one mesocycle, or month, at a time rather than trying to simultaneously develop different abilities.[162] In a trial comparing periodized with non-periodized strength training, the periodized group showed improved maximum performance after four and eight weeks, while the non-periodized group showed no improvement even after 12 weeks of training.[163]

Another study of trained exercisers compared a group doing four weeks of plyometrics followed by four weeks of no plyometrics with another group doing seven straight weeks of plyometrics. Both groups gained strength equally, but the seven-week plyometric group seemed to obtain little additional benefit from their three extra weeks of plyometrics. Following the period of intense plyometric exercise with four weeks of recovery, interestingly, was just as strongly correlated with gaining strength as was doing the exercise itself.[164] In a related study, a 5.4 percent decline in jump performance was observable after seven weeks of heavy strength training, but changing the training regimen – to four weeks of ballistic jumping –
not only reversed the decline but caused a rebound that in some cases exceeded the athlete's start-of-season performance.[165] These studies suggest that periodization works and indicate that emphasis on intensifying techniques like ballistic loading or plyometrics might be optimized by placing them within a periodization design using month-long blocks.

But what's the best way to incorporate cardio into the workout blueprint? Strength and cardio seem to oppose each other: after all, you run slower after a bout of strength training and you can't do as many push-ups after a hard run. This interference between cardio and strength is documented by studies showing that strength training done too soon before cardio training does dampen cardio performance,[166] and that cardio training dampens at least some aspects of strength performance, especially for the muscle groups directly involved in any preceding cardio exercise.[167] While you can occasionally combine both types of exercise in the same session and still get strength and cardio-related improvements,[168] habitual concurrent strength and cardio training sessions eventually compromise strength and muscle development, perhaps from the cumulative effect of inferior strength performance from tired muscles. The performance lag was seen to last for as many as eight hours, affecting whatever type of work, whether cardio or strength, that was performed second in the workout session.[169] So if you do perform strength and cardio work in the same session, you might want to place whichever type of training at which you most want to improve first in the session. Athletes usually separate their strength and cardio sessions by at least a few hours,[170] and if you follow the training routines in this book, you will, too, most of the time. We'll usually be keeping strength and cardio workouts themselves separate – except for Routine 6, "Tough," and Routine 8, "Plyo," which deliberately require you to do strength and cardio concurrently, alternating bursts of strength and cardio activity over the course of a three-mile run.

If you're considering dodging the interference effect by doing a month of only cardio or only strength training, it might be helpful to know how long you can go doing one kind of training before losing the benefits specific to the other. Studies suggest that once your muscles are trained, you could go as long as an entire month without strength training and experience minimal atrophy and strength loss.[171,172] You lose the effects of cardio training somewhat more quickly, with aerobic fitness losses appearing in less than five days.[173]

It also may help in your planning to recall why you're doing strength and cardio training in the first place. If you primarily want to lose fat, you'll want to emphasize cardio, because, as we have seen, it burns calories. Only cardio exercise typically produces weight loss,[174] perhaps because of the tremendous potential for calorie loss from sustainable repetitive movement like jogging. During cardio work, time flies and the calories burn: an intriguing study compared the calorie cost and perceived effort of 30 minutes of cardio cycling with 30 minutes of squat strength training using weights. It found that the cardio, which burned 442 calories, was rated as easier than the squat training, which burned only 269 calories.[175] To the extent that losing fat is your priority, the cardio-intensive workouts of Routines 3, 6, and 9 are the ones to look at for providing training that emphasizes burning calories.

Yet cardio training alone won't change your proportion of fat to muscle, or body composition: if you're a fat apple (android) or pear (gynoid), cardio might only make you a smaller apple or pear. For most people, a "skinny fat" physique that technically fits into the desired clothing size but has drooping rolls of fat is not the ideal outcome of a fitness program. To get a "V" shape, with big shoulders and strong legs, you'll want to do strength training, which may not by itself appreciably reduce the amount of fat you carry but does change your body composition by increasing the size and amount of lean muscle.[176]

Even when emphasizing strength training, try to always retain some form of cardio, such as the modest 45 minutes of daily exercise recommended by the United States Surgeon General,[177] or the three days a week of cardio thought to be the minimum needed to avoid gaining fat along with muscle.[178] A way to do this is to limit cardio to a number of sessions per week low enough so that whatever your goal, whether it is to do strength training three, four, five, or six times a week, not a single session of strength training is missed because you were too tired from doing cardio. The routines in this book help this happen by having you usually alternate strength days with cardio days. In one of the few studies to recommend actual day-per-week frequency, a review noting the benefits of strength training on older adults suggests you might benefit by limiting cardio to three days per week during periods in which you are seeking to maximize strength gains.[179]

It is probably not useful to persist with doing strength training at one level obsessively to the exclusion of others, and better to use periodization to systematically pursue endurance, strength, and speed. Try to move beyond just building strength endurance to include more challenging speed and power activity like ballistic loading and plyometric movement. Perhaps due to disuse, fewer fast muscle fibers survive into advancing age than slow-twitch fibers, and a relative absence of fast-twitch fibers constitutes a primary difference between old and young muscle.[180] Pursue vigorous strength activity beyond just building endurance to hold on to your fast-twitch muscle fibers and keep them active. Don't make the mistake many bodybuilders do by overemphasizing upper body strength work, with the unfortunate result of an intimidating upper body but skinny legs. Keep leg strength exercise prominently in the picture, as do the training routines in this book. In a study looking at most of the data on aging and muscle, loss of muscle function at about five percent per decade was noted to begin after age 40, to affect fast-twitch fibers more than slow-twitch fibers, and to involve muscles of the legs more than muscles of the arms.[181]

A lot of periodization schemes micromanage training with microcycles, undulating periods, linear progressions, and alternating light and heavy workouts, but research comparing such complex periodization schemes has not found any one design to be clearly superior to any other.[182] In two studies of trained exercisers, steady progression resulted in greater gains in strength than up-and-down hard days alternated with easy days.[183,184] Perhaps the best advice is do not get entangled in microcycles and undulating light and heavy days, but try your best each time you work out.

The periodization method this book uses is a simple three-month cycle that gradually shifts from building endurance and stamina in the first month, to developing strength in the second, then maximizing power and speed in the third. Periodization also solves the problem of the contrasting, even opposing nature of the different fitness domains, a workout design problem that becomes more pronounced as you become better trained, as long strength workouts with their heavier workloads are harder to combine effectively with short, intense speed or power workouts, just as peak strength training and cardio experiences rarely happen together. As you gradually achieve higher levels of endurance, strength, or speed, planning one kind of workout that lets you continue to get improvement in all three different domains gradually becomes a problem. The only way to get really good at doing opposing types of exercise is to focus on each type of training at different times. We'll use the three-month cycle as a simple but flexible template to build endurance, then strength, then power, season after season, setting you on a path to improvement that still leaves room, as you will see, to vary and individualize.

Periodization also prevents the stagnation and decline that follows overly monotonous training. Even with gradual intensification, repetitive workouts eventually lead to diminishing returns. The obvious sign that you might be overtraining is if a feeling of staleness, fatigue, and irritability replaces the high you usually get from working out: a review of studies on overtraining concludes that its clearest manifestation is mood change.[185] Another indication that you might be overdoing it is if you come down with a cold, or, as researchers call it, an upper respiratory tract infection.[186] Despite the increased risk of catching a cold during periods of heavy or intense training,[187] exercisers in general get fewer of them,[188] and once you have one, doing exercise neither shortens nor prolongs a cold's duration.[189,190] The fascinating *Ah-Choo! An Uncommon History of the Common Cold*, summarizing the otherwise rather inconclusive state of current research on colds, suggests we think of them as opportunities for respite: "Maybe it's a good thing to be laid up once in a while, compelled by nature to shift our routine and retreat from everyday pressures."[191]

It's likelier for most of us to suffer more from under- than over-training. Resting, after all, is easier than exercise, and it's human nature to default to comfort instead of make an effort. Exercise requires a conscious choice. Perhaps having a lackluster workout now and then due to overtraining might be worthwhile insofar as regular workouts build a valuable tendency to habitually exercise. Only if you have been doing regular heavy exercise might tapering down the volume (the total amount of time spent exercising) or even taking a few days off towards the end of a three-month cycle help you fully realize and even augment its benefits.[192]

Yet constant change need not be a rigid, uncompromising regimen of periodized workouts. Change can be as small as trying a new exercise or as large as skipping strength training for a while to do only cardio. Vary your exercise to keep it interesting. Within the confines of common sense, the workout routines in this book will serve you best if you occasionally bend them or even set them aside, and then, refreshingly, return. If you have time, sample different fitness disciplines like tai chi, yoga, or weight training, or get involved in sports like soccer, rugby, or basketball. Even moderate physical activities like gardening, golf, housework, or walking have their own benefits. Feel free to shake things up, knowing that this book's training program is always here for you.

With these seven steps of fitness, you now know something about how to get the most out of your workouts. The structured routines in this book attempt to put this advice into action, to provide a logical and thorough way to express much of your genetic potential for fitness, starting with endurance, work tolerance, and discipline; then intensity, strength, and neuroendocrine response; and finally, speed and power before returning again to endurance. You'll be using the cyclic progression method that athletes use, building higher-performance and more intense movements on a base of endurance. The law of specificity that dictates that the best way to get better at a specific task is to practice doing exactly that task, used in the sports industry to grind athletes into a pencil-point of hyperspecialized competitiveness, works here in your favor to methodically build up your performance across an array of very different physical pursuits. While strongmen become bigger and distance runners become thinner, you will become a little bit of both, or more simply put, you will grow healthier. This book uses a cycle not to push yourself into specialty, but to bring out your whole genetic potential by forcing you to work on your weakest areas as well your strongest. Every workout in this book involves endurance cardio, every workout requires strength and speed. If you have a gift, the workouts you're about to do will give you opportunity to use it, but they will also help develop your weak areas, too. Making you deal with each of the three fitness domains – endurance, strength, and speed – cyclic progression solves fitness problems. Hate running? The cycle gives you plenty of opportunity to finally begin to enjoy it – but without taking you away from strength-building exercises. Don't even like the sound of speed strength training? In this book, the road to power and plyometric work is paved with longer, mellower workouts that you might fall in love with. Whatever your genetic predisposition, the three-month cycle of body-weight exercises in this book range across a robust spectrum of land-based movement from the slow and steady to the quick and powerful in order to bring out your best in all the fitness domains. It is harder to develop your weaker areas than to specialize in your strongest, but in doing so, you'll not only become fitter in the truest and most well-rounded sense of the word you will learn, I think, something of what makes life worthwhile.

Let's put these principles into practice with workouts you'll find easy to learn and remember.

Section 2

THE
WORKOUTS

e'll look at four workouts, each based on a fundamental human movement. The four workouts involve 42 different exercises, separated into pushing, lifting with your legs, pulling, and running. Start with a warm-up, such as running to the location where you're going to exercise, or lightly perform related preliminary movement, like jumping jacks (page 38) or windmills (page 42); a recent study, echoing others, found that warming up resulted in measurable improvement on 79 percent of fitness performance criteria.[193] Try to work out every day, alternating strength days with cardio days, or even double up, if and when that works for you, by doing strength training in the morning before breakfast and cardio in the afternoon before lunch or dinner. Use the workouts to make a routine of your own, or choose from the 11 routines that come next.

Keep your technique simple, intuitive, and unforced. In general and unless instructed otherwise, breathe out with the effortful part of the movement, which is when you push, lift, jump, or pull during a strength exercise. Returning to the neutral or starting position comprises the less effortful part of the movement, and is when you should breathe in. Don't obsess about perfect form. Try to keep your body weight centered, your head and shoulders up, and your back erect, not rounded or slumped forward. When doing the strength exercises that involve leg movement, try to lift with your legs and not your back. You can find your way to better form by remembering to breathe out during the effortful part of the movement, opening up your chest, and keeping your weight centered and balanced on your feet. When doing cardio, focus primarily on covering the distance goal you've set yourself, and letting your own best technique emerge naturally.

For each of the four workouts, I will explain how to do the primary exercise, why the movement is useful, how to make it easier or harder, and how to take the primary exercise further with related exercises. To make learning easy, each workout lists its exercises, with a few necessary exceptions, in alphabetical order.

WORKOUT 1:
PUSH

All the exercises in this workout come from one movement, pushing with your arms. You push when you lift heavy objects above your shoulders, raise yourself up from a bed or chair, or push yourself away from objects or the ground. Starting with the push-up, a familiar workhorse, these exercises will develop your chest, shoulders, and triceps with air boxing, clap push-ups, dive bombs, grounded dips, jump outs, jumping jacks, plyometric jump outs, plyometric push-ups, side bridges, triceps push-ups, and wide push-ups.

primary exercise **Push-up** Get into position by squatting down and placing your palms on the ground shoulder-width apart in a comfortable position. Jump back, extending both legs straight back (if 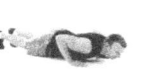 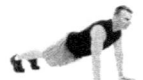 that's too hard, bring one leg back at a time). You now should be supporting your body weight on your palms and the balls of your feet, with your feet and legs close together, and your legs and trunk forming a straight line going up from your feet to your head. Several of the exercises in this workout start with this posture, which is called "plank position." To do the actual push-up, lower yourself down so your chest touches the floor, then push your entire body up from the ground, pushing through your hands, breathing out as you go up. Keep your back relaxed but straight.

WHY Long the exercise of choice for assessing and developing upper body endurance, the time-honored push-up loads your upper body, chest, triceps, forearms, trunk, and abdominal muscles. The number of push-ups you can do serves as a simple test of overall fitness: the top 10 percent of men in their twenties can do at least 42 push-ups in a row; for women, that figure is 32. The average man in his twenties can do 24 push-ups in a row, the average woman in her twenties, 16. But roughly the same numbers apply to only the fittest 10 percent of men and women in their sixties.[194] To the extent they provide beneficial mechanical stress to your bones, push-ups help maintain healthy cartilage and bone. While men have long used push-ups as upper-body muscle builders, women like how push-ups tighten and tone their upper body and triceps.

EASIER Because the push-up puts more than a quarter of your body weight on each wrist, people with wrist or shoulder pain may find a regular push-up hard at first. If you feel shaky, or have persistent trouble keeping your back straight, lighten the load by letting your knees rest on the ground. If that's still too hard, do wall push-ups, which are the same as regular push-ups, except that you stand up and push against a wall. Most people can do wall push-ups without aggravating their wrist or shoulder pain. To make the wall push-ups gradually harder, gradually step farther back from the wall to so that you have to lean more to do the push. In time, with regular workouts, you'll be able to work up to knee push-ups, and then to full-fledged regular ones.

HARDER The simplest way to make push-ups harder? Do more. Military recruits routinely show up for training able to do 100 push-ups in good form without stopping, well above the 42-push-up norm for the top 10 percentile of males in their twenties. As you become able to do more push-ups without stopping, apply the intensification techniques of working to failure (page 23), continuous movement (page 26), muscle targeting, or ballistic loading (both on page 27).

PUSH EXERCISES The 11 push exercises each stress different muscles in different ways. In addition to push-ups, choose at least three of these that seem to work for you. Use the same guidelines for these exercises as you did for push-ups, training first for endurance, then intensifying.

1. Air boxing Assume a boxing stance: bent elbows and clenched fists (with your thumbs over, not inside, the fingers). Keep your forearms close to your abdomen and a little open so that the palm part of your wrist is up (like when pitching underhand softball) and your pinky fingers almost touch the sides of your torso. Punch out one arm 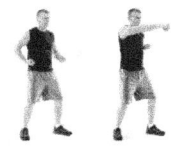 as hard as you can and retract it. As you retract one arm, punch out hard with the other, punching an imaginary spot in mid-air. As you punch, let your wrists corkscrew 180° so the punch ends with your knuckles forward and on top.

2. Clap push-up (You should be able to do at least 20 push-ups in good form, without wrist pain, before attempting a clap push-up.) 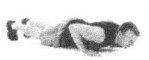 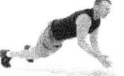 Perform a push-up, pushing up with an extra thrust so you can clap your hands together before landing. The clap should be distinctly audible. Like with any challenging movement, introduce this exercise cautiously, and only when you think you're ready.

3. Dive bomb   These push-ups load up a broader area of your chest and shoulders. Assume the plank position, but with your hips up in the air so you're bent at the waist in a V shape, with straight legs and straight arms. Keeping your hips high, lower your chest to the ground in between your hands. Continue forward, pushing your chest through your hands and then up, straightening your arms so that your hips are now down and your head and shoulders high. Now go in reverse back to the starting position. Breathe evenly as you do this, don't cheat by holding your breath.

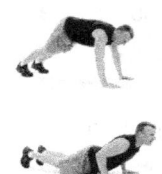
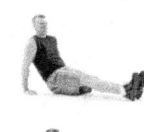

4. Grounded dip   Assume a forward sitting position, sitting with your legs relaxed and in front of you, knees slightly bent. Place your hands comfortably at your sides to support yourself. Use your legs and abdominals to hike your hips and rear end off the floor so that you're balancing on your heels and hands. Now lower yourself by bending your elbows just enough so your rear just touches the ground, then straighten your elbows to raise yourself back up to complete one grounded dip.

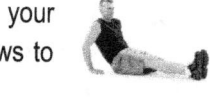

5. Jump out   This vigorous five-part movement, also called a "burpee," oscillates between a crouch, a plank, and standing. Start by crouching down

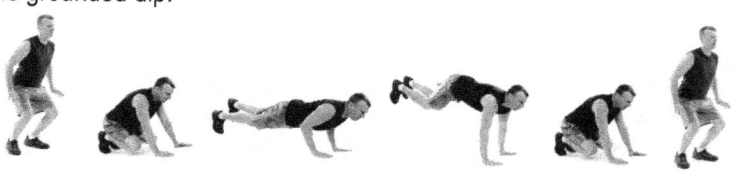

and placing both palms on the ground shoulder-width apart. Jump out to extend both legs straight back so your feet land behind you, then fast as you can, jump in to return both feet back to the starting position. Your palms stay in place until you are finished, when you jump back up to standing.

6. Jumping jack   Stand with feet together and arms down. While sweeping your arms sideways and up over your head, jump and open up your legs to land on the ground with your feet roughly shoulder-width apart. Throughout the movement, keep your legs straight, but your elbows should be slightly bent in a way that feels comfortable. This transition movement (which you might remember from gym class) can give you a break before the next plyometric exercises.

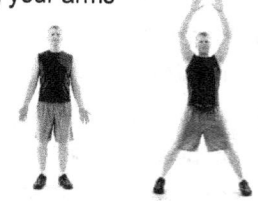

7. Plyometric jump out   Try this only after you are somewhat trained, so don't attempt this until you can do five clap push-ups – and you shouldn't even try a clap push-up until you can do 20 regular push-ups without wrist pain. This is a jump out without the squat: you jump and thrust your legs back in mid-air to land on your palms. Begin by standing with knees and elbows slightly bent, palms outward. Now jump up and lean forward and down to land on your palms and the balls of your feet, absorbing some of the landing impact by bending your elbows as you would in a push-up. You should land in a posture about midway between the start and end of a push-up. Pushing with your arms, jump quickly forward into a crouched position and leap back up as quick as you can, knees lining up over, not in between, your feet as you complete the quick return to standing.

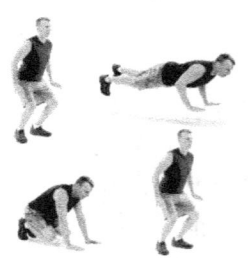

8. Plyometric push-up You should be able to do five clap push-ups before attempting this. Start in a high kneeling position, with your trunk and thighs standing vertically. With palms out, ready to brace you, fall forward and land on your hands. Let your elbows bend with the impact to 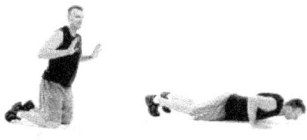 absorb some of the shock, and let the rest of the shock stretch your chest and triceps muscles. The moment you land, push hard with your arms to propel you back up to the starting position.

9. Side bridge This is a sideways push-up. Prop yourself up sideways and balance your weight on your right arm and the side of your right foot. Now bend your right elbow to lower yourself as far as you can, 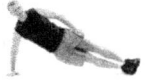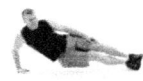 and straighten it to push yourself up. Like grounded dips, this exercise targets the triceps muscles and provides beneficial load-bearing stress to your shoulder, elbow, and wrist joints. It also requires a great deal of balance. Repeat the set with your left arm.

10. Triceps push-up Start in plank position, but with your hands close enough together to form a triangle, your thumbs and index fingers touching. Narrowing your base of support forces the 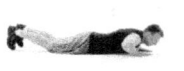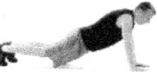 load on your triceps as well as your inner chest muscles. Bending your elbows, lower yourself so that your face nearly touches the ground. Push up by straightening your arms, as in a normal push-up.

11. Wide push-up Start in plank position, but with your hands far apart, so that your upper arms are almost straight out to the sides. Lower yourself until your chest just touches the ground, 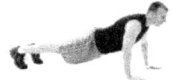 then push up until your arms are straight. These exercises can be hard on your shoulder ligaments, so do them cautiously at first until you're used to them. Push up from the center of your body, using your chest more than your arms.

WORKOUT 2:
LIFT

One of life's most basic actions, lifting yourself with your legs, often neglected by typical exercise programs, is the challenging primary movement of this workout. Although people use their legs every day, they train them less than any other muscle group. The human body seems to have the genetic potential for approximately twice as much leg as arm strength, as suggested by world records for strength, yet the legs of even highly trained exercisers are often only marginally stronger than their arms.[195] Legs also seem to not only tolerate but thrive on heavier exercise than arms. In one study comparing single-set and three-set strength training, the two extra sets resulted in a superior adaptation for leg strength, but not for arm strength.[196] In a follow-up study, the extra-two-set protocol was again compared against doing one set and again found to provoke a heightened gain in strength and in size for legs more than for arms.[197] In a third study, adding in ballistic training increased absolute maximum leg strength, as measured by the one-repetition-maximum squat, more than merely performing heavy squatting alone, and this ballistic-related strength gain for legs also was substantially more than that observed for arms.[198] A fourth study showed that four sets produced superior strength gains in the legs compared to one set, and eight sets were better than four: the still higher number of sets did not lead to an as-expected diminished return due to exhaustion but instead, still greater strength gains.[199] Leg strength also closely relates to fall risk in older people: the presence of gait or balance abnormalities increases fall risk by three times, but leg muscle weakness increases it by five times.[200] Because of such evidence in favor of substantial leg strength training, plenty of leg exercises appear in all the workouts, but this particular one focuses on legs entirely and on using them to carry out a most important body movement – lifting your body weight against gravity. Leg power contributes to all body movement, so these exercises will improve your trunk and upper body performance as well. Your leg muscles are your largest, and include the biggest (the gluteus maximus) and longest (the sartorius) muscles, so although the exercises are harder, they also use more calories and result in greater absolute strength than upper body exercises.

primary exercise **Deep squat** Place your feet in a stance that feels comfortable and natural to you. Bend your knees and lower yourself down. Avoid tipping forward by letting your sitting bones move back, keeping your weight over your feet and your heels on the ground. Think of yourself as pushing your feet against the ground as you lower yourself as far as possible while keeping good balance. Then slowly lift yourself back up.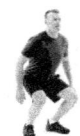

Form – how well you balance yourself – is important here. Many people, including experienced exercisers, do not squat properly. Some cheat by not bending their knees all the way or not putting their legs into it, missing the full benefit of this movement; others incorrectly let their knees approach each other. So let's review perfect form. Keep your head and shoulders up, and curve your back, letting your hips go back and your knees bend. Balance solidly over your feet, keeping your knees over your feet and not over the ground between your feet. While keeping your head erect and shoulders back, allow your rear to go backward. Moving this way is natural and has several benefits: it puts the heaviest load where it belongs, on your large quadriceps muscles, not your knees; it protects your lower back by accentuating its normal curve; and it keeps your center of gravity over your feet. Go slowly, feeling your leg muscles really working, and stay in control, because bouncing at the bottom of the movement can hurt your leg muscles or knee joints. Keep your heels on the ground and your knees over and not inside of your feet. Lower yourself until your thighs are parallel to the ground before you start to lift yourself back up. As you return to standing, push with your feet. Exhale as you push up from the soles of your feet, driving the movement from your feet to maximize the engagement of your leg muscles. Using good form like this is also an example of the intensification technique of muscle targeting (page 27).

WHY The deep squat satisfies three criteria of an ideal exercise: it's a big movement, it's weight-bearing, and it's closely related to real-life activity. All effective leg-training workouts include some form of the squat. Because it works out all of your leg and trunk muscles in one exercise, squats are tiring, but they efficiently work many large muscles at once in both the lifting and the lowering movements, burn more calories per minute than easier exercises, and also load and strengthen the cartilage, joints, and bones of your back, hips, knees, ankles, and feet.

EASIER Anyone with knee, hip, or back pain may find squats hard, but if you get out of bed, raise yourself up from a chair, or climb out of a car, you do squats already. You just have to make this particular squat a little easier. Don't lower yourself as far down as possible, only to the point that is ever so slightly more uncomfortable than you think is okay. Then straighten back up. Or, if you need to, start by leaning against a wall to take some of the weight off of your knees. As long as including the modified squat in your training still challenges you, you'll not only get stronger, but also find everyday tasks, like moving from bed to chair or from sitting to standing, gradually getting easier. If you've never done squats before, wait to see how you feel the next day before going all out with a large number of repetitions. Muscle soreness means you should wait a day before repeating squats, and because it can peak a day or two after the workout, it's commonly called "delayed onset muscle soreness." As hard as it may be to believe, exercise – although at reduced intensity and duration – might be the best way to deal with muscle soreness.[201] While it's normal to feel sore in your muscles after using your lower- body muscles for squats for the first few times, if your joints feel hot or swollen after exercise, you're doing too much. As with any other exercise, don't make it too difficult too quickly; give yourself the weeks of time, if necessary, that you might need to get used to heavier exercise. In time, you will be able to work up to doing a session or two each week of squats that go very deep without the aid of a wall. Take the time you need to develop a stable, deep squat without having to move fast or lurch forward to complete the movement. As you work, you'll also be getting into the habit of doing an exercise essential for lifelong fitness.

HARDER Regardless of your training level, a properly performed deep squat is a significant loading event and a potent stimulus to develop lean muscle. Build endurance first, by doing more repetitions and more sets of repetitions. Then try the intensification techniques to which squats lend themselves particularly well: continuous movement, muscle targeting, ballistic loading, and plyometrics. For continuous movement, drop the pauses at the top and bottom of the movement, changing the 10 repetitions into one long motion. At the top and bottom of the movement, don't pause so much as instantly change direction, but still always keep the movement steady, controlled, and slow. Still too easy? Use muscle targeting by continuing to improve your technique, but go slower to make the squats harder. Relax the muscles as you are sinking down, consciously letting go of any tension in your lower body, while at the same time keeping the movement steady and slow, even very slow. As you rise up, exhale but stay relaxed and controlled. You will feel a heavy load on your leg muscles as you straighten up. Or use ballistic loading to "bounce in the middle" by shortening the range of movement and increasing speed. For a greater challenge still, try the last five of the 11 leg exercises, which are all plyometric movements.

LEG EXERCISES These leg exercises each derive from the squat movement, although the last five, the plyometric exercises, are in a class of their own. The leg exercises all develop your lower body strength and power: contact squats, forward lunges, gentle jumps, karate kicks, rear lunges, one-leg squats, plyometric jumps, plyometric jump variations, lunge jumps, and bounds and hops. In addition to squats, find at least three of these exercises that work for you. The leg exercises may seem a little more difficult than some of the other exercises, but leg strength is a critical fitness attribute over the lifespan. As you get older, you'll miss having your former leg strength more than you'll notice losing arm strength.

1. Contact squat   From a standing position, squat all the way down. Place your palms on the ground, knees touching the insides of your arms, supporting your body weight on the balls of your feet and hands, and let your heels rise slightly as you look forward. Quickly return to standing.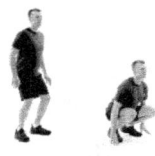

2. Forward lunge   The lunge is as fundamental a lower body strength developer as the squat, so try to include this exercise consistently. Beginning from standing, step forward with your right leg as far you can without losing balance. Bend your knee to lower yourself down deeply but comfortably. Begin to push off even as you hit the lowest part of the movement, breathing out with the effort, returning to starting position. Repeat with the left leg. (While it's faster to just do many repetitions with one leg and then the other, take the time to change stance and alternate each repetition with a different leg. Changing stance improves your coordination and ensures that you train both legs equally.)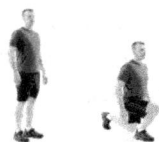

3. Gentle jump   Start from standing and lower yourself partway into a squat, then jump up and forward slightly. This modified version of the jump puts beneficial loading stress on your pelvis, hips, knees, ankles, and feet, which will prepare you for the explosive forces generated in plyometric jumping.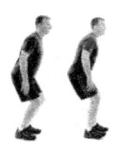

4. Karate kick   Stand solidly on the ground, elbows bent slightly, with your right leg planted slightly behind your body. Pivoting on your left leg and rotating left, bring your right leg forcefully forward. Bring your bent right knee across your center to the left, and explosively extend your right foot out and to the front. Return to starting position, repeat for each repetition of the set. Do same for left leg.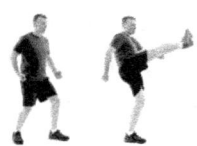

6. One-leg squat   Balance your body weight on the right leg and lower yourself into a squat, as far as you can. Exhale as you straighten back up, and focus on keeping your balance. Repeat with the left leg. This exercise is difficult, but with time, you eventually should be able to lower yourself so that your thigh is parallel to the ground, while keeping good form (head erect, back straight, center of gravity over base of support, and heel on the ground). If this is too hard, modify the movement by letting the opposite forefoot lightly touch the ground.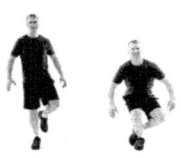

5. Rear lunge   Standing with your feet shoulder-width apart, take a giant step back with the right leg, touching down with the ball of your foot. As your foot touches, continue to lower your body, feeling the stretch in your hip and trunk. Return to starting position. Repeat with your left leg.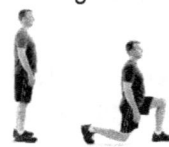

PLYOMETRIC EXERCISE: ARE YOU READY?

The next five leg exercises use plyometric movement to develop your lower body strength and power. Plyometric exercises are hard, but you can and should use them, as long as you've developed a good base of strength and conditioning by practicing the preceding leg exercises first. Before trying plyometric exercise, see if you can:

- three one-leg squats in which the weight-bearing thigh comes almost parallel to the ground without any pain or difficulty,
- five clap push-ups, and
- one 100-yard sprint at your perceived maximum speed.

If you have to modify how you do any of the above, then you have to likewise modify how you do plyometrics. The idea is to push yourself with what you have, but not so hard that you get hurt.

7. Plyometric jump Start from a standing position, lower yourself as rapidly as you can into a full squat, knees always over feet (if you were to look down, you should always be able to see your big toes), and jump explosively upward as high and fast as possible. To increase your jump height, reach up with both hands as you ascend. As you land, sink back into a squat to repeat the exercise.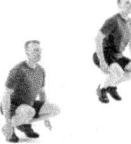

WHY By putting your body under a unique combination of stresses, plyometric jumps stimulate a unique combination of adaptations. During the loading phase of a plyometric movement, your muscles and the connective tissue around them store energy by stretching quickly, like a spring. As you jump up, forward, or outward, an inborn stretch response reflex helps you recoil explosively. These movements build strength and resilience by reinforcing muscle, tendon, ligament, and bone. Each plyometric exercise relates closely to real-life activities like jumping, running, striking, or throwing, and they quicken the righting responses that prevent you from falling when you've been thrown off balance. Plyometrics may even, as discussed on page 28, improve your running economy. Unlike the close relationships between many of the exercises we've looked at and the improvements they confer, the benefits of plyometric movement seem to be broadly based.

EASIER By definition, doing plyometric movement slowly means it's no longer plyometric, and, moreover, you also lose the assistance of your stretch response reflex if you do the exercise too slowly. If you need to make a plyometric movement easier, shorten your range of motion instead. Bend only until it's slightly uncomfortable, and gradually deepen the movements over the course of different sessions until you can do them more fully.

HARDER As with other strength exercises, to make the plyometric movements harder, just do more of them. Gradually add more repetitions per set, or more sets, or both. Plyometric work is measured in foot contacts, or how many times you land during a session. As you get stronger, you can make an entire session out of the different plyometric exercises, totaling 80 to 120 foot contacts. Athletes using plyometrics routinely perform sessions involving up to 300 total foot contacts. As an alternative, you can shorten the usual two-minute rest period between sets.

These last four exercises both require and develop explosive strength.

8. Plyometric jump variations: forward, zig-zag, and sideways (You should be able to do plyometric jumps before doing plyometric jump variations.) Instead of jumping straight up, jump forward with each jump, jump diagonally, zigzagging 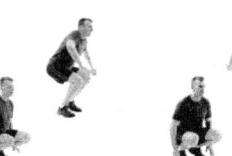 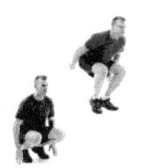 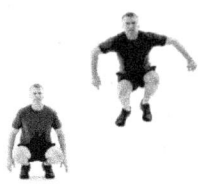 back and forth, or jump sideways. Each of these variations in direction stresses a different set of muscles. You can emphasize height, by hanging in the air as long as possible, or distance, by trying to make each jump longer than the previous one.

9. Lunge jump (You should be able to do plyometric jumps before doing lunge jumps.) Start with a lunge stance, one leg forward and one leg back, but with your pelvis still facing evenly forward. Lower yourself about two feet, then jump explosively, as high as you can. Switch your legs in midair, landing with the other leg forward.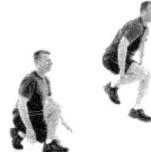

10. Plyometric jump variations: knee-tuck and pike (You 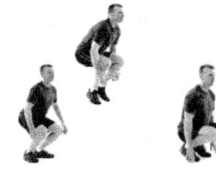 should be able to do plyometric jumps before doing plyometric jump variations.) To do a knee tuck, start from standing, lower yourself to a squat, and then jump as high as you can. Tuck both your legs as high as possible, pressing them to your chest by quickly grasping your knees. Release in time to land. To do a pike, lift your legs as you jump, trying to both straighten your knees and touch your toes with your hands before landing.

11. Bound and hop (You should be able to do plyometric jumps before trying 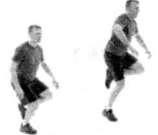 bounds and hops.) While jumps use both legs in unison, bounds and hops use just one leg. A bound means leaping off with one leg and landing on the other, just as you do in running. A hop, on the other hand, means landing on the same leg that you leapt with. With each bound or hop, try to maximize forward distance, air time, and speed, moving forwards as quickly and quietly with the largest movements you can make while still maintaining control. Explosively fire the springs in your legs to get as far forward as you can with each bound or hop, land quietly and efficiently so as to quickly bound or hop forward again.

Having finished the strength workouts, we turn now to the most frequent workout you will do, Workout 4, "Run." It will show you a range of cardio exercises, from simple walking all the way to activities like interval training, speed drills, and sprints so intense that they could also be described as strength training. Except for swimming, all exercises in Workout 4 relate to the body's most basic task: movement across land.

WORKOUT 3:
PULL

This workout develops your ability to pull, using your upper body to lift objects to you or to pull up your body weight while hanging from something you grip with your hands. Some of the exercises – the pull-up, hanging knee raise, straight-arm pull, underhand-pull-up, and wide-grip pull-up – require a bar, which you can often find in your neighborhood park or recreation area – you can even use a jungle gym. Or you can get a pull-up bar that fits into a doorway without hardware on Amazon for less than $70. Any stable, sturdy horizontal bar or pipe that can support your weight and from which you can hang from comfortably and safely will do. The remaining pull exercises – the bend and reach, cobra stretch, extend and flex, forward bend, high jump, and windmill – further engage your back, biceps, rear shoulders, and core.

primary exercise **Pull-up** Grasp a bar with an overhand grip (palms facing 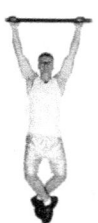 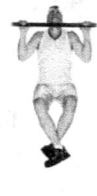 forward). You might find your grip stronger and more sustainable if you place your thumb alongside the knuckle where your index finger meets your hand (instead of wrapping your thumb around the bar). That way, your thumb muscles are working alongside your forearm grip, not in opposition to it. This "ape" version of the overhand grip works especially well on the thicker bars that you typically find available outdoors, but on thinner bars, the conventional opposing-thumb version of the overhand grip works better (with this grip, wrap your thumb around the opposite side of the bar so that your hand forms a cylinder). Use whichever overhand grip works best for you. To execute the pull-up, hang from the bar and pull your body upwards as high as you can. Pull yourself up smoothly, without wrenching or swinging. If you swing, you're cheating with momentum from your hip muscles, instead of fully using your back. Try to pull high enough to squeeze your shoulder blades together and get your chin over the bar. Lower yourself with control so that you don't swing.

WHY Pulling, the second fundamental upper body movement, is required for climbing, bringing objects closer to your body, and lifting your body up with your arms. The pull-up develops the latissimus dorsi muscles, or "lats," which are the upper body's largest muscles, as well as many neighboring muscles all along the back and arms, including the biceps. A simple and respectable (if monotonous) routine would be to do 50 pull-ups, resting as many times as you need. Being able to do eight pull-ups in a single set is a good early benchmark; people in peak condition can do 25 or more in a row. It takes more upper body strength to perform a pull-up than a push-up. Some people may not be able to perform even one pull-up, but by modifying the movement as described below, you can build up to doing one pull-up. Once you can do one, you're on your way: by working at sets of one, you can gradually build up to sets of two, then three, then five, and so on.

EASIER Increase your pulling strength by doing straight-arm pulls or by getting assistance from a partner or a push-off surface, like a sturdy box, crate, or platform. The straight-arm pulls, described below as one of the related exercises, strengthen the muscles used to initiate pull-ups. A partner could help you by grasping your sides just above your hips and giving you only enough of a boost to help you complete a pull-up without swinging or jerking. Alternatively, you can use a solid box or push-off surface to help you, combining the pull-up with a push-off from the surface with your feet.

HARDER Besides doing more repetitions, you can make pull-ups still harder by resting for a shorter time between sets, or by performing them more slowly. Make sure, though, that you pull your chin all the way up past the bar every time.

PULL EXERCISES The 10 remaining pull exercises include the hanging knee raise, straight-arm pull, underhand pull-up, and wide-grip pull-up, which also require a bar, and the bend and reach, cobra stretch, extend and flex, forward bend, forward jump, and windmill, which don't. Try to include some bar exercises, as they will strengthen your forearms as well as your back. Don't worry about forcing yourself to get your chin up high over the bar every time, just try to do as full and complete a movement as you can. If no other bar exercise seems possible, start with the hanging knee raise and straight-arm pull. These develop your ability to hold onto the bar and will over time enable you to do a half and eventually a full pull-up.

1. Hanging knee raise Hanging from a bar using the same overhand grip as you did for the first pull-up exercise in this workout, with your legs fully extended, raise your knees to your chest. Lower them in a controlled motion. This exercise uses your forearms and wrists as well as your abdominals. Like the straight-arm pull exercise that comes next, it's also a great way to develop your ability to hold onto the bar, laying the foundation for performance gains in the other bar exercises.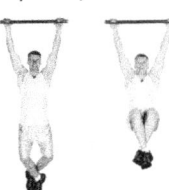

2. Straight-arm pull   This exercise targets the muscles that stabilize your 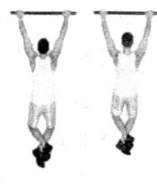 shoulders and builds strength to help you do full pull-ups. Hanging from a bar with an overhand grip (palms facing forward, as you did during the first pull-up exercise), retract your shoulder blades to bring them together, pulling yourself upward using your shoulder and upper back muscles. Remember to keep your arms straight. Relax the muscles in your shoulder blades to slowly return to starting position.

3. Underhand pull-up   A "underhand grip" means that your palms are 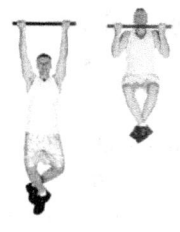 facing you when you grab the bar. This pull-up puts the focus on your biceps and wrist flexors. Grasp the bar, pull yourself up, get your chin over the bar, and lower yourself back down without swinging. If you are working on a thick bar, you may need to use a mixed grip, which means you would stand with your torso perpendicular, not parallel, to the bar. When you grab the bar with a mixed grip, one palm faces right, one palm faces left, and you pull yourself up alongside the bar, alternating on the right and left sides.

4. Wide-grip pull-up   Wide-grip pull-ups emphasize the lower part of your 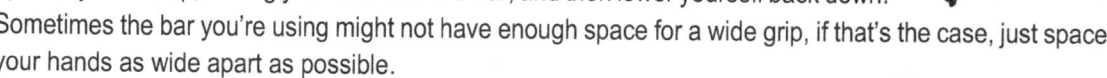 lats. Grasp the bar with your hands wider apart than you would do for a regular pull-up. Pull yourself up, raising your chin over the bar, and then lower yourself back down. Sometimes the bar you're using might not have enough space for a wide grip, if that's the case, just space your hands as wide apart as possible.

5. Bend and reach   Standing with your feet shoulder-width apart, lift your 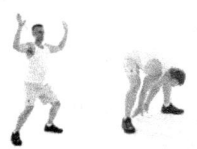 arms straight overhead, then swing your arms down, and squat as you bend forward at the hips. Reach backward between your legs, keeping your arms straight and your heels on the ground. Swinging your arms back and up over your head, return to standing.

6. Cobra stretch   This easy stretch is good for a tight back. 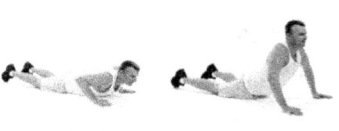 Lying on the ground prone (on your stomach), place your hands by your shoulders and push-up until your arms are straight, but relax your spine so that your belly sags gently towards the ground. Breathe out as you relax your belly.

7. Extend and flex   Start in the plank position, with your weight 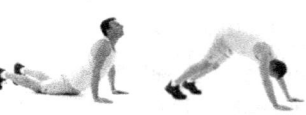 on your palms and the balls of your feet, and with your spine, legs, and elbows straight. Let your torso sag and look up while you exaggerate the normal curve of the small of your back to let your belly dangle without allowing your knees to rest on the ground. Then reverse the position, and stretching your back and leg muscles, arch your back like a cat so much that your heels lower until they nearly make contact with the ground. Return to the starting plank position. This movement, which you may recognize as the cobra and dog stretches from yoga, prepares you for the exercises that come next. This is a good time to talk about yoga and exercise. Yoga means unlocking your inner physical potential by linking — "yoking" — together mind, body, and soul. In classical yoga, the pelvic area is called the *mula bandha*, the root lock. You can think of this extend and flex movement as a way of unlocking the root lock, as a way of attaining unity of mind, body, and soul.

8. Forward bend   Stand, bend forward from your hips, as though they were a hinge. Try to bend as far forward as you can, bending your knees only slightly, then use your back muscles like pulleys to straighten yourself back up slowly. Forward bends put some load on the joints of your spine, so as with all exercises, give it a try but also respect any sharp pain as your signal to modify or stop the movement.

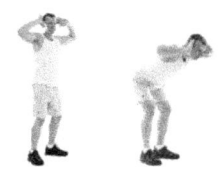

9. Forward jump   Do this gently at first if you're not used to vigorous exercise. Start in a forward-leaning position: knees slightly bent, trunk leaning forward, with your arms stretched behind you in line with your torso. Swing your arms forward and upward, and jump forward as high and far as you can. Then swing your arms backward and jump back. As you lean forward, bend from your hips, but do not slump or round your back: your torso should be in a straight, forward-leaning line.

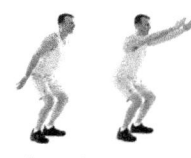

10. Windmill   Stand with feet shoulder-width apart, arms outstretched to each side. Touch your right hand to your left foot, bending forward at your hips and only slightly at your knees. As you do so, rotate left, pulling your left arm back to keep both arms straight. Return to starting position, and repeat with the left: touch your left hand to your right foot, bending your hips and knees to rotate right. As you bend, pull your right arm back to keep both arms straight. Return to starting position.

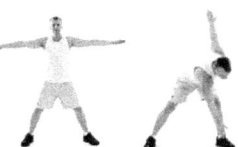

WORKOUT 4:
RUN

The first three workouts train for strength, but this one takes place on the other end of the fitness spectrum, using steady-state and higher-intensity forms of cardio to focus on locomotion across land. While discussing cardio, we'll cover not just walking and jogging – and how to enjoy them, no matter what your fitness level – but also running, speed training, and sprinting, all ways your body efficiently executes its oldest task: travel.

With a treadmill or access to a large indoor space, such as a mall, atrium, or an indoor track, you can do this workout inside, and because there's no equipment required, you can also do it outside. The outdoors offers more interesting visuals, as well as fresh air, and a growing array of lightweight clothing makes exercise comfortable in all kinds of weather. Whatever your speed or mode of locomotion, the whole world is out there for you to move around in. Get the most from this workout by going for distance, layering up in cold weather, and protecting your skin from sun and friction.

- *Go for distance, not for time.* Choose a favorite path to walk or jog, maybe through a park or around a scenic part of your neighborhood, and complete that route every day. Work up to traversing one mile, two miles, or even three or more. First build your endurance, gradually lengthening your workout while keeping the intensity low, only later gently introducing bursts of higher speed. Take your time. Learn not just how to tolerate the exertion, but also how to enjoy these long, low-intensity sessions. After all, you're trying to forge a habit that will last a lifetime.

■ *Layer up on the extremities, less around the core.* To trap more body heat to stay comfortable in cold weather, use multiple light layers instead of one heavy coat. Wear one layer less than you would if you weren't exercising, to allow for the extra heat generated by exercise. If you feel a little chilly during the first few minutes, you're dressed properly. Don't skip gloves or a hat; a lot of heat escapes from your hands and head. In time, you will adapt to be more comfortable in all kinds of weather. Even heavy rain or snow doesn't need to stop you. In time, only extreme heat (above 100° F with high humidity), cold (below 15° F with high wind), or lightning ("When thunder roars, go indoors") need prevent you from enjoying exercise outside.

■ *Don't burn, don't chafe.* With the ozone layer still thinning, ultraviolet radiation levels and skin cancer risks continue to rise. To avoid damaging your skin and aging it before its time, protect exposed skin with a sunscreen with an SPF of at least 15. Protect the retinal lining of your eyes from UV rays with sunglasses. If you need to, avoid inner thigh chafing by applying a petroleum jelly such as Vaseline or wear compression undershorts before you go out for a long period of running or walking.

The first exercise, walking, prepares you for jogging, hiking, and the heightened activity level so important in burning fat. More active people may wish to skip ahead to jogging, introduced next, but if you're new to exercise or have any doubts about whether you will enjoy regular jogs, build a foundation for effective cardio workouts by starting with walking.

primary exercise **Walking**   Take a walk. Observe your posture as you begin: are you standing straight up, but relaxed? Square your shoulders and move them back to open up your chest. Move your head back, too: over half of us have a forward head posture, an understandably common condition, given that so much that compels our attention – the book, the computer, the desk, the television, and the windshield – is situated directly in front of us. Simply straightening up eliminates the slouched, rounded shoulders that often accompany forward head posture. Stand tall, then relax slightly into a better posture. (Since our bones change shape under mechanical stress over the years, an upright posture might feel strange to you. Keep reminding yourself to straighten up, square your shoulders, and move your head back. Over time, better posture will become easier as your bones continue to remodel.)

Now that you're standing straight (but not rigidly straight), take a deep breath from your diaphragm, the large sheet of muscle that runs under your rib cage. Sigh the air out fully without forcing it. Forceful or overly deliberate breathing engages other rib muscles that can interfere with the diaphragm's job. Holding in your abdominal muscles also interferes with breathing. Instead, let your belly relax as you inhale. Relax as you exhale, too, to efficiently expel air by letting your diaphragm resume its comfortable domed resting shape. By improving your posture, relaxing the rib cage muscles, and letting your diaphragm muscle work for you, you've just increased your lung ventilation by almost a third, and reduced your systolic blood pressure by a measurable amount as well. In yoga, breathing fully from the diaphragm in this manner is called *ujjayi*, or "the victorious breath," and it will calm you. Even as your body's other respiratory muscles – located along your neck, ribs, and abdomen – begin to kick in during the labored breathing of exercise, you should let your breathing come from the diaphragm.

With this natural, diaphragm-driven breathing in place, you're ready to enjoy walking. Relax your arms as you walk, letting them swing forward. We can think of walking as emerging from a complex combination of interactions. Your embedded motor control system takes into account the unique elastic and mechanical properties of your body, simultaneously and subconsciously adjusting your contact with the ground. These behind-the-scenes motor operations do not limit you, they guide you. Like a pendulum finding its equilibrium, as you keep moving, you find the most efficient pattern of movement for any given speed of locomotion, and much of this discovery happens without your conscious effort. Your job is just to keep moving forward at your chosen speed.

WHY Of all the exercises in this book, walking is the single activity that can be done by the greatest number of people for the longest length of time. A 170-pound person on an easy stroll burns six calories each minute. While six calories may not seem like much, walking is one of the few exercises enjoyable enough to be sustainable over many minutes and many years. Walks help you lose fat and prevent rebound weight gain, as they did for 82 dieters doing regular exercise walking.[202] Walking powerfully intervenes against high blood pressure, a precursor to the common conditions of cardiovascular disease, diabetes, and obesity that pervade in our sedentary society, as evidenced by a study in which just a moderate 1.86-mile daily walk by itself significantly reduced high blood pressure.[203] Your walks will particularly benefit you as you get older: because walking builds bone mass, lifelong walkers experience a far lower risk of hip fractures,[204] a significant cause of death in advanced old age. Walkers also suffer less dementia, or mental confusion, during their later years.[205] Pleasant, weight-bearing, and available to almost everyone, walking helps develop the endurance, neuromuscular control, and strength necessary for the other exercises in this book.

EASIER Walking may be the gateway to all the other exercises in this book, but it isn't always easy. If it's hard for you, take heart: your walking capacity grows every time you walk. Develop a habit of regularly walking however far you can comfortably go. Identify how far that is – Four blocks? One block? Down to the corner? – and resolve to walk that distance every day, plus just a few steps more. Then keep adding a few more steps every day. Stretch your limits a little and walk just a bit farther than what's comfortable, and feel good about what you've done that day. With proper rest and nutrition, your body will adapt to this gradual, gentle overload by growing stronger. Eventually, what was uncomfortable will be comfortable, and the daily walk that was short will be long. It will get much easier, if you give it time and stick with it. In my practice, I've spent a considerable amount of time motivating people to walk, and some have shared what has worked for them to get more walking into their lives. Here are some of the best:

"Wake up a little earlier than usual and go for a walk before breakfast."

"Choose a slightly longer walking route to your car, work, or house."

"Try not to think about it – just put on your shoes and go, remembering that the walk will boost your alertness and energy."

"Find a favorite quiet street or park far away enough to be a good walk or run to get to, and visit it routinely."

"Go outside for a walk at least once a day, no matter the weather."

HARDER   While a great exercise habit to start with, walking remains a relatively modest form of cardiovascular activity. Jogging delivers all the benefits of walking in half the time, and provides additional beneficial aerobic and weight-bearing stress. Even if medical problems like arthritis, joint pain (especially in the shoulder, knees, or back), heart trouble, diabetes, or obesity make jogging seem like a daunting prospect, it still may be within your reach with this slow, safe method:

THE ONE-MINUTE-A-DAY RUNNING METHOD

- *First time, one minute.* For your first jogging session, start with five minutes of walking, and then take a jog for only about a minute. Keep it to just one minute of jogging, and devote the rest of the time to walking.
- *One more minute each day.* For the next jogging session, add on just one more minute.
- *Keep at it.* If you have a day where jogging just doesn't work for you, try again the next day. What seems like too much one day will be easier the next. Don't give up.
- *Assess.* As you progress toward a full workout session spent jogging, ask yourself how you are doing. It's normal to feel a little sore afterwards, especially at first, but keep in mind that symptoms like night pain, pain with every step, or any kind of persistent discomfort might signal a problem. If the symptoms do not go away with rest, call your doctor.

The one-minute-a-day method lets you ease slowly into jogging. If you are wary of it, take as much as a year of slow, steady sessions, and mix intervals of walking and jogging to work up very gradually to a pure jogging session.

CARDIO EXERCISES   Compared to walking, the benefits of jogging are an order of magnitude greater. Before going on to the more challenging activities of interval training, speed drills, sprints, hiking, and swimming, let's take a closer look at jogging.

1. Jogging   Good jogging begins with you remembering what you may already know, then forgetting it. Start with an upright but comfortable posture. Your head should not sway or jut forward. Stay vertical, relaxed, and stable. Let your arms swing forward and backward, without sideways movement, neither going below the midline of your body nor swinging higher than armpit level. Neither your hands nor teeth should clench. Each foot should land quietly. Think instead about the midpoint in your pelvis between your two hip bones. Imagine that it is tied to an invisible rope pulling you forward. Don't pound the ground with your feet, but land lightly, letting the rope pull you. Mentioned in the work of Dr. Moshe Feldenkrais, founder of the therapeutic exercise technique that bears his name, this concept of pelvic drive has helped people run with greater enjoyment and better performance.[206] Now relax, let go of holding onto perfect posture and work instead on sustainable speed. As during walking, your brain works behind the scenes to achieve maximum efficiency at whatever speed you choose, and does this work even better without your conscious interference.

Jog as fast as you can comfortably. You don't need to push for a painfully high speed. If you enjoy your jog, you're more likely to keep doing it, and such persistent exercise over time will outweigh any benefits from an exercise program that you quit. The perfect equilibrium at which your muscles take in oxygen without accumulating lactic acid, called "steady rate," happens at a comfortable pace. If you speed up to an uncomfortable or painful pace, your body shifts from steady rate to a high-intensity anaerobic metabolism that, while helpful for other kinds of conditioning, won't sustain you over the long workouts needed to meaningfully improve your endurance. An Iowa State University study of 30 individuals jogging at increasing speeds confirmed that onset of displeasure coincided with the shift from aerobic to anaerobic metabolism. The authors of the study suggested that jogging as fast as you can while still finding it pleasurable was the best way to keep jogging sessions long-lasting enough to maximize their aerobic benefit.[207] So whether you jog a mile in 12 minutes or in eight, unless you are specifically working on speed training, create a lasting habit by usually going only as fast as you can enjoyably.

WHY Jogging offers a faster, better, and more sustainable way to burn fat. As mentioned on page 16, you burn 40 percent more calories per mile by jogging rather than walking, and you cover the same mileage at least twice as quickly, if not more. Since you can burn calories so much more quickly while jogging, this highly efficient exercise should be the calorie-burning method of choice for most busy people. Moreover, each jog produces incremental improvements in speed and ease of movement. Jogging perpetuates itself: the more often you use this powerful method to burn energy, the better jogger you will become.

How much jogging can people do? A lot. A National Runners' Health Study surveyed 8,283 recreational runners and concluded that the more people jogged, the more health benefits they accrued. Although increasing mileage beyond 50 miles a week continued to bring additional benefits, the rate of improvement diminished,[208] and for men, remember that as mentioned on page 24, running more than 40 miles per week associates with decreased testosterone.

EASIER How fast you can go depends on your fitness. There's nothing wrong with jogging slowly. If you're just starting, particularly if you're overweight, jogging might not be the right activity for you – yet. Instead of forcing yourself, use the slow, safe one-minute-a-day method described earlier to transition from walking to jogging. Go for a sustainable lifelong habit, not just a few spectacular workouts finishing in a flameout. Be patient. Go as fast as you can while still enjoying it, even if that means walking. You'll still be burning calories and improving your fitness. Nothing wins out over persistence.

HARDER As you adapt, you'll want to keep your jogs interesting by increasing the distance you run or by gradually speeding up the pace. Try to extend your distance, or cut your time, by increments of 10 percent. By increasing your pace, you force your body to burn food energy more efficiently. Just keep in mind that like any constructive overload, a faster jogging pace is difficult, and may be somewhat uncomfortable at first. Hills, steps, and stairs offer other ways to intensify, as do the remaining cardio exercises in this workout. If you live near a stadium, you can intensify your jogging by going up and down the steps. For example, the little South Boston soccer stadium amphitheater in my neighborhood has 11 sections of 15 11-step aisles each, enough for a 20-minute workout if one runs up or down each aisle. Jogging uphill is obviously more work, but jogging downhill also helps force coordinated movements at a faster speed to let you experience a higher stride frequency than you could otherwise achieve. It also increases eccentric load, or the work your muscles do while lengthening. Just make sure the slope is not so steep that you find yourself landing on your heels to brake. Make sure you can land on the ball of your foot, the part which normally makes contact with the ground first. Going farther or faster, downhill or uphill, on stairs or on steps – these are all ways to make your jog more challenging.

Think of jogging as mainly an aerobic activity. That is, it develops oxidative capacity and promotes endurance. As we've seen, your best strategy for finding your optimal training speed is by jogging just under the threshold of discomfort. However, as you continue training, you also will be doing intervals of higher-intensity anaerobic running during which your muscles will be burning fuel too fast for immediate oxygen replenishment. This kind of running uses an entirely different metabolic pathway than that relied on by jogging. During such anaerobic, or speed training, your body turns to muscle sugar and other non-oxygen-supplied fuel, and engages the stronger and thicker fast-twitch muscle fibers that are specialized to perform without immediate need of oxygen replenishment. Interval training, speed drills, and sprints deepen and extend your cardio workout, training you for speed, while hiking and swimming offer alternatives to running.

2. Interval training   Alternating jogging with higher-speed runs or sprints pushes you to perform better, fatigue less, and run faster with less lactic acid buildup. This not only improves your ability to tolerate

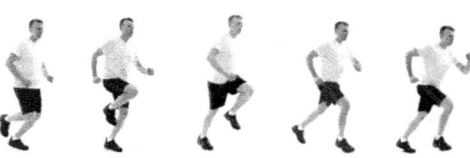

bursts of speed, but also raises the pace at which you can comfortably sustain a prolonged jog. These five interval training exercises let you acclimate to intensities too extreme to sustain over an entire workout. Usually the harder activity alternates with intervals of the easier in a 1:2 ratio, like the six cycles of 60-second sprints and 120-second jogs used to train military recruits. However, for more strenuous activity such as sprinting, the rest interval can be longer, shortening only as you become better trained. (For example, the one-minute-a-day method back on page 50 coaxes walkers into running with a harder-to-easier ratio of 1:19.) Most digital watches have stopwatches you can use to time the intervals, but you can also mark off intervals using only your instinct. Run quickly until you simply can't anymore, and then go back to jogging until you feel ready for another bout. Or, run your intervals on a track to give you a precise idea of the distances that you are covering. Here are five exercises in interval training:

- *The 1:2.* Perform the harder activity for one minute, and then let yourself recover by doing the easier activity for two minutes. Repeat seven times for a 21-minute workout.
- *The 1-to-5.* For this tough but brief 20-minute session, think of "1" as the easiest level of activity, and "5" as the hardest level. The hardest level for novices may simply be walking as quickly as possible, for example, while for conditioned athletes it may mean sprinting at top speed. For the first minute, do a "1." The next minute, do a "2," and so on, until you're doing a "5" (your most strenuous exercise) in the fifth minute. Repeat this cycle four times, for a total of 20 minutes. Keep this exercise highly structured by measuring the minutes with a stopwatch (available on most digital watches), or choose landmarks spread about a minute apart as goalposts. Although straightforward, the 1-to-5 is not easy!
- *The 4-by-4.* The innermost lane of standard tracks is a quarter-mile long, four laps makes a mile. Run two laps, jog one lap, repeat three more times for a total of four cycles or 12 total laps. Work towards completing the entire three miles in 30 minutes or less while emphasizing speed for the laps you run but allowing a slower recovery pace for the laps you jog. A track

lane converter (page 61) shows how to run the same mileage in track lanes other than the innermost lane. Another way to do the 4-by-4 is to run four cycles of four minutes at or close to your highest sustainable level of effort followed by three minutes jogging at a recovery pace, for a total of 28 minutes. Either way, the 4-by-4 develops aerobic capacity, or $VO_{2\,max}$, an important indicator of fitness and conditioning.

- *The Long 12.* The straightaways on all standard track lanes are 92 yards (84 meters) long. Using any track lane, run six laps, jogging the curves and sprinting the straightaways for a total of 12 sprints. The emphasis of this exercise is on achieving faster sprint times, as long as you still maintain an actual jogging pace on the curves. If you use the innermost lane, you run a total of about one-and-a-half miles, half the distance of the preceding 4-by-4 exercise, and if you run in an outer lane, you run slightly more distance (up to 14 percent more) on the curves and with proportionately longer jogs between sprint bouts.

- *The Short 12.* Identify a 35-meter (38-yard) distance, such as between the touchdown and 6 feet short of the 40-yard line on a football field, or a little less than half (41 percent) of the 84-meter-long straightaway on a standard track. Sprint the 35 meters, rest 10 seconds as you walk back to the start, and repeat for a total of 12 sprints. With a little practice, you can use the stopwatch function to time the sprints. Keep your turnaround walks under 10 seconds long. If you cut this drill in half (to six sprints), you'd have the Running-Based Anaerobic Sprint Test (RAST) on which this drill is based. The RAST is used to develop and to test anaerobic capacity, an important indicator of power and ability to perform explosive movement in basketball, football, hockey, rugby, and soccer.

SPRINT WITH COMMON SENSE

Mindful of the possibility of causing you to collapse on the track, I hasten to add that you should not literally sprint at your highest theoretically possible speed, as if being chased by a cougar. Even superbly conditioned athletes sprint at about 85 percent of their theoretical maximum.[209] Most people who try to run all out or as fast as they can will approach this 85 percent maximal speed, but your sprinting speed should be tempered by consideration of your body, your age, your conditioning level, and common sense.

3. Sprints When you sprint, you try to run as fast as you can, about 85 percent of your maximal possible speed. Sprinting uses an astonishing amount of energy, another order of magnitude greater than that used by jogging. While jogging uses 40 percent more energy per minute than walking, an all-out sprint uses 360 percent more. Sprints, like other intense training activities, raise your metabolism by burning additional energy even after the activity is completed, as evidenced by measurements showing that just a single bout of sprinting increased total daily energy expenditure by about 10 percent.[210] Sprinters also develop tremendous strength – as a look at the legs of an Olympic sprinter would seem to confirm. Sprints are often done in football-field lengths of about 100 yards, or you can also train for shorter or longer distances. Of course you'll get better mainly at the type of sprint you practice consistently, with longer sprints expanding your endurance and aerobic capacity, while shorter, faster sprints will develop a somewhat different capacity for muscle strength and power. Sprinting is magical: like no other exercise, in sprinting, one grasps, for a moment, the infinite.

4. Speed drills   If you already run perfectly, the best speed training might be to simply to run a familiar distance faster. However, most of us have a weak component in our running pattern. To find it, try each of the following drills that runners use to improve their speed. Choose the one that seems the hardest to do – the drill during which you have the most trouble achieving and keeping good form. By working on your weakest point, you can bolster your overall performance and the stronger components of your run so that your running can achieve greater economy. Of course, you may find as you advance that you have a new weak point relative to the rest of your abilities; if so, shift focus accordingly.

- *Foot turnovers.* This drill speeds up your running cadence. Leaning against a wall or ledge, lift and bend your knee up, then push it down, out, and around in a circle while keeping it bent, as if you were riding a bicycle. Start slow and work up to completing the circle as fast as you can. Repeat for the other leg.

- *Laterals.* Laterals use your hip muscles to improve your balance. Begin by standing slightly crouched, your feet shoulder-width apart and your head up. Step sideways by bringing the trailing leg to the lead leg, and quickly hop to the side to land back in a crouch with your feet shoulder-width apart. Repeat to move sideways as quickly as you can, picking the feet up with each step and keeping your hips low but back straight. Avoid knocking your ankles together.

- *Verticals.* Verticals improve your running form. Exaggerate normal running form, bringing your knees forward and up to waist level, bending your legs to a 90° angle from your torso. Swing the opposite arm forward with each raise of the knee. (When your right leg is forward, the left arm is forward and the right arm swings back.) Keep a strong, smooth arm swing, with your lead forearm also bent to 90° and rear arm nearly straight. Your arms should swing front to back, not side to side. Keep a tall stance and a stable, upright torso. Move as fast as you can with good balance. If it doesn't flow, slow down.

5. Hiking   Now we come to my favorite activity of them all, hiking. All you need is comfortable clothing and shoes, good weather, and, depending on where you're going, appropriate insect countermeasures. A diverting alternative to flat-terrain running or walking, hiking combines lower-intensity strolling with spurts of higher-intensity travel on uneven terrain. It also provides many new challenges. Walking over sand takes nearly twice as much energy as traversing solid ground, and soft snow takes three times as much. Also, the varied terrain of hiking requires you to step in a coordinated manner so as not to trip or turn your ankle on the uneven surface, a skill you might want to develop gradually with short hikes. Hiking warrants caution, common sense, and a partner, but it refreshes the spirit as well as the body. As conservationist John Muir better put it, "Climb the mountains and get their good tidings. Nature's peace will flow into you as sunshine flows into trees. The winds will blow their own freshness into you, and the storms their energy, while cares will drop off like autumn leaves."[211] Research corroborates Muir's enthusiasm: lower body fat and blood pressure, smaller waist circumferences, reduced cholesterol, and improved moods were all still measurably evident in hikers some seven weeks after the end of a three-week daily hiking program, according to a study of Austrian vacationers.[212]

6. Swimming With its movement cushioned by water, swimming complements running. The most efficient swim stroke is the front crawl, also called "freestyle": swim horizontally, reaching each arm alternately forward to enter the water, catch it, pull back, and release out of the water (led by the pinky-finger side of your hand). Let your body rotate slightly back and forth with the alternating arm cycle, along the long axis from your head to toes, staying streamlined to reduce the water's drag. Kick with your whole leg, not just from the knees, to stay in slipstream, keeping your kick mostly underwater and no more than about seven inches deep. Breathe bilaterally to the side of each arm as it releases out of the water to facilitate even technique, or unilaterally if it's more comfortable for you, always exhaling underwater. Find a marvelous discussion of swimming techniques in Steve Tarpinian's excellent *The Essential Swimmer*.

The Routines

We've looked at 42 exercises grouped into four workouts. The next 11 routines fit these workouts into training programs accommodating a variety of schedules and skill levels, starting with a beginner's routine for the novice exerciser. They also bring you into a three-month cycle that will systematically progress from endurance to strength, speed, and performance using six routines each devoting half a month to progressively harder intensification techniques, of doing 300 repetitions, working until failure, continuous movement, muscle targeting, ballistic loading, and plyometrics. Three alternate routines, one for each of the three months, allow emphasis on successively more intense forms of cardio. Finally, as promised, there's a routine asking busy people for no more than 20 minutes, three days a week for strength exercise. Always check with your physician before beginning an exercise program, and use common sense when choosing a routine or progressing its intensity.

This three-month cycle is easy to remember and puts you in synch with the seasons if you start it on the first day of January, April, July, or October. If you first start in mid-season, you might like to lengthen or shorten your first cycle in order to start the next cycle on one of those days. This seasonality can give cadence to a satisfying rhythm of activity, with the three-month cycle wrapping up near celebratory times like spring break, the longest days of summer, peak autumn, and end of year.

Of course, some of us prefer no routine at all. If this is you, make your own strength workout by choosing at least three different strength exercises, doing at least three sets of eight to 20 repetitions apiece for each exercise, alternate every other day with one or two cardio activities like walking or running for as long a distance as you comfortably can, and occasionally combine strength and cardio in concurrence in the same workout.

Let's get started!

ROUTINE 0: WORKOUT ZERO

Each workout in this routine will take about 20 minutes to do. If any of the exercises in this or any other of the workouts seems too hard, modify them as you like to make them easier. A workout that you enjoy is a workout that you can sustain. As this routine gets, well, routine, start adding the exercises under "add" to make each workout roughly 10% harder each week and begin adding distance to your mile-long jog, as well as working on running faster.

Monday
WORKOUT 1: PUSH
push-up 10, 10, 10
air boxing 20, 20, 20
grounded dip 10, 10, 10
jumping jack 10, 10
side bridge 10, 10
triceps push-up 10
wide push-up 10
add
dive bomb 5, 5, 5
jump out 5, 5, 5

Wednesday
WORKOUT 2: LIFT
deep squat 10, 10, 10
contact squat 10, 10
forward lunge 10, 10, 10
gentle jump 10, 10, 10
karate kick 10, 10, 10
rear lunge 10, 10
add
contact squat 10, 10
one-leg squat 5, 5

Friday
WORKOUT 3: PULL
hanging knee raise 10, 10
straight-arm pull 10, 10
bend and reach 10, 10, 10
cobra stretch 10
extend and flex 10, 10
forward bend 10, 10
windmill 10, 10
add
pull-up 5, 5, 5
forward jump 5, 5, 5

Every day
WORKOUT 4: RUN
1-Miler: walk and jog 1 mile, starting by jogging 10% of the mile the first week, 20% the second week, and so on

ROUTINE 1: 300

Build endurance strength by doing these strength workouts, which each total 300 repetitions (page 22), and running three miles for cardio. Do this routine the first half of the first month of your three-month cycle. Ambitious exercisers can double up this or any other routine by doing the strength workout in the mornings Monday through Saturday, and the cardio in the afternoons, Sunday through Friday.

Monday
WORKOUT 1: PUSH
push-up 35, 25, 20, 20
air boxing 30
clap push-up 5, 5, 5
dive bomb 10, 10, 10
jump out 20, 10
plyometric jump out 5, 5, 5
plyometric push-up 10, 10
side bridge 20
triceps push-up 10, 10
wide push-up 20

Wednesday
WORKOUT 2: LIFT
deep squat 20, 20, 20, 20, 20
contact squat 20, 20
forward lunge 10, 10, 10, 10
gentle jump 20
karate kick 10, 10, 10
one-leg squat 5, 5
rear lunge 10, 10, 10
plyometric jump 10
lunge jump 10
knee-tuck jump 10

Friday
WORKOUT 3: PULL
pull-up 10, 10, 5, 5, 5
hanging knee raise 10, 10, 10, 10
straight-arm pull 10, 10, 10, 10
underhand pull-up 5, 5, 5, 5
wide-grip pull-up 5, 5, 5, 5
bend and reach 30
cobra stretch 5
extend and flex 20
forward bend 30
forward jump 10, 10, 10, 10
windmill 20

Tuesday, Thursday, and Saturday
WORKOUT 4: RUN
Long Run: run as far as you can, at a comfortable pace, going for the longest overall distance (at least 3 miles) you can cover in an hour, trying to get used to jogging the same route

ROUTINE 2: WORK

This routine asks you to repeat each movement until you can't do a single additional repetition in good form. The number next to the exercise refers to how many sets of repetitions you do until achieving momentary failure – the temporary inability to continue the movement with perfect form (page 23). Alternatively, complete a total number of repetitions of each exercise equal to the total number you did for the previous routine plus one more (that number is in parentheses). Do this routine in the second half of the first month.

Monday
WORKOUT 1: PUSH
push-up 3 (101)
air boxing 2 (31)
clap push-up 2 (16)
dive bomb 2 (31)
jump out 2 (31)
plyometric jump out 2 (16)
plyometric push-up 2 (21)
side bridge 1 (21)
triceps push-up 2 (21)
wide push-up 2 (21)

Wednesday
WORKOUT 2: LIFT
deep squat 3 (101)
contact squat 2 (41)
forward lunge 2 (41)
gentle jump 1 (21)
karate kick 2 (31)
one-leg squat 2 (11)
rear lunge 2 (31)
plyometric jump 1 (11)
lunge jump 1 (11)
knee-tuck jump 1 (11)

Friday
WORKOUT 3: PULL
pull-up 4 (36)
hanging knee raise 3 (41)
straight-arm pull 3 (41)
underhand pull-up 3 (21)
wide-grip pull-up 3 (21)
bend and reach 1 (31)
cobra stretch 1 (6)
extend and flex 1 (21)
forward bend 1 (31)
forward jump 3 (41)
windmill 1 (21)

Tuesday, Thursday, and Saturday
WORKOUT 4: CARDIO
Timed Long Run: run the same 3-mile route,
your best pace, trying to shorten your time

ROUTINE 3: RUNNING MACHINE

As often happens in life, this alternate routine for the first month mixes cardio and strength concurrently, with an emphasis on running. On Tuesday, Wednesday, and Friday, run as efficiently as you can, but stop to do a single set of the specified repetitions of a strength activity in good form, then spring up to quickly resume efficient running.

Monday
WORKOUT 4: RUN
on the first day, run as far as you can in 1 hour, for the rest of the month, repeat the distance, and once you can do it comfortably, work on running the route in 90, then 80 percent of your original time

Tuesday
WORKOUT 1: PUSH and WORKOUT 4: RUN
run same route you ran Monday, combine with
push-up 35, 20
dive bomb 10, 10
jump outs 10, 10
plyometric push-up 10, 10

Wednesday
WORKOUT 2: LIFT and WORKOUT 4: RUN
combine Monday's run with
squat 20, 20, 20
forward lunge 10, 10
karate kick 10, 10
plyometric jump 10

Thursday
WORKOUT 4: RUN
warm-up jog for 2 minutes, then
interval training: the 1:2:
run at high speed for 1 minute,
jog comfortably for 2 minutes,
repeat 7 times for 21 minutes

Friday
WORKOUT 3: PULL and WORKOUT 4: RUN
combine Monday's run with
pull-up 8, 5, 5, 5
wide grip pull-up 5, 5
forward jump 10
windmill 20

Saturday
WORKOUT 4: RUN
warm-up jog for 2 minutes, then
The 1-to-5: starting easy, run 5 minutes, each minute at a faster pace, repeat 3 times for 20 minutes

ROUTINE 4: CONTINUOUS

Minimizing rest between sets and within repetitions, this routine ups the intensity to make each strength workout ideally a long continuous movement (page 26). Try to eliminate pauses within each strength movement, and limit rest between sets to less than a minute. Running up and down hills or stadium steps is not only symbolic and inspirational, it develops aerobic capacity. Do this routine the first half of the second month.

Monday
WORKOUT 1: PUSH
push-up 20, 19, 18, 17, 16
air boxing 75
clap push-up 7
dive bomb 12
jump out 12
plyometric jump out 7
plyometric push-up 10
side bridge 20
triceps push-up 10
wide push-up 10

Wednesday
WORKOUT 2: LIFT
deep squat 40, 39, 38, 37, 36
contact squat 15
forward lunge 15
gentle jump 20
karate kick 10
one-leg squat 5
rear lunge 15
plyometric jump 10
lunge jump 10
knee-tuck jump 10

Friday
WORKOUT 2: PULL
pull-up 10, 9, 8, 7, 6
hanging knee raise 10
straight-arm pull 10, 10, 10
underhand pull-up 7
wide-grip pull-up 7
bend and reach 20
cobra stretch 5
extend and flex 20
forward bend 10
forward jump 15
windmill 20

Tuesday, Thursday, and Saturday
WORKOUT 4: RUN
Stadium Steps: run 2 miles up stadium steps or up hills at your best pace

ROUTINE 5: TARGET

These strength sessions are shorter and more intense. Do each movement listed in **bold type** slo-o-o-wly and deliberately using the muscle targeting technique (page 27) to achieve temporary exhaustion at the end of each set, so that you truly cannot do one more rep. The track lane converter below shows the equivalent total distance for this or any other running session when using other than the innermost lane. Do this routine the second half of the second month.

Monday
WORKOUT 1: PUSH
push-up 20, 15, 10, 10
dive bomb 10, 10, 10
triceps push-up 10, 10, 10
wide push-up 10, 10, 10

Wednesday
WORKOUT 2: LIFT
deep squat 20, 20, 20
forward lunge 10, 10, 10
karate kick 10, 10, 10
one-leg squat 5, 5, 5
rear lunge 10, 10, 10

Friday
WORKOUT 3: PULL
pull-up 10, 10, 5, 5, 5
hanging knee raise 10, 10, 10
straight-arm pull 10, 10, 10
underhand pull-up 5, 5, 5
wide-grip pull-up 5, 5
forward bend 20
windmill 20

Tuesday, Thursday, and Saturday
WORKOUT 4: RUN
The 4-by-4: on the innermost lane of a track, run 4 cycles of 2 fast laps, 1 slow for a total of 12 laps, or 3 miles, in 30 minutes or less, or off track, run 4 cycles of 4 minutes fast, 3 minutes slow

TRACK LANE CONVERTER: RUNNING THE OUTER LANES

	WIDE-STANDARD TRACK, WITH 48-INCH (1.22-METER) WIDE LANES			NARROW-STANDARD TRACK, WITH 42-INCH (1.07-METER) WIDE LANES			
LANE	% OF LANE 1	2-MILE DISTANCE, IN LAPS	3-MILE DISTANCE, IN LAPS	% OF LANE 1	2-MILE DISTANCE, IN LAPS	3-MILE DISTANCE, IN LAPS	LANE
1	100%	**8.0**	**12.0**	100%	**8.0**	**12.0**	1
2	102%	**7.8**	**11.8**	102%	**7.9**	**11.8**	2
3	104%	**7.7**	**11.6**	103%	**7.7**	**11.6**	3
4	106%	**7.6**	**11.3**	105%	**7.6**	**11.4**	4
5	108%	**7.4**	**11.1**	107%	**7.5**	**11.2**	5
6	110%	**7.3**	**11.0**	109%	**7.4**	**11.1**	6
7	112%	**7.2**	**10.8**	110%	**7.3**	**10.9**	7
8	114%	**7.0**	**10.6**	112%	**7.2**	**10.7**	8

ROUTINE 6: TOUGH

Think you're tough? This alternate routine for the second month returns to concurrent strength and cardio training and trains you on two **bolded** basic tasks: doing least 35 push-ups in good form and running two miles in less than 16:36. Mondays, Wednesdays, and Fridays, run 3 miles, stopping every 500 feet or so to do a strength exercise, on the other days, improve your 2-mile run speed. (To run two miles in other than the innermost lane of a standard track, use the track lane converter on the previous page.)

Monday
WORKOUT 1: PUSH and WORKOUT 4: RUN
combine 3-mile run with
push-up 35 or more
air boxing, 100
clap push-up 10
dive bomb 20
jump outs 20
jumping jack 50
plyometric jump out 20
plyometric push-up 20
triceps push-up 20
wide push-up 20

Wednesday
WORKOUT 2: LIFT and WORKOUT 4: RUN
combine 3-mile run with
deep squat 50
contact squat 30
forward lunge 20
karate kick 20
one-leg squat 5
rear lunge 20
plyometric jump 10
forward jump 10
bounds 20
hops 20

Friday
WORKOUT 3: PULL and WORKOUT 4: RUN
combine 3-mile run with
pull-up 10, 10, 10
hanging knee raise 20, 20
underhand pull-up 10
wide grip pull-up 10
bend and reach 20
extend and flex 20
windmill 20

Tuesday, Thursday, and Saturday
WORKOUT 4: RUN
2-Miler: 8 laps around the innermost lane of a track at 16:36 or faster
and, on Tuesday
WORKOUT 3: PULL
pull-up 10, 10, 10
and, on Thursday
WORKOUT 1: PUSH
push-up 35 or more

ROUTINE 7: BALLISTIC

Apply ballistic loading, the technique of moving quickly back and forth without pause within the middle range of the movement (page 28), to the **bolded** exercises. This routine, for the first half of the third month, introduces timed sprints into the cardio workouts.

Monday
WORKOUT 1: PUSH
push-up 30, 20, 20, 20
air boxing 150
clap push-up 5, 5, 5
dive bomb 10, 10
jump out 20, 10
plyometric jump out 10, 10
plyometric push-up 10, 10
side bridge 20
triceps push-up 10, 10
wide push-up 10, 10

Wednesday
WORKOUT 2: LIFT
deep squat 20, 20, 20
contact squat 20, 20
forward lunge 10, 10, 10
gentle jump 20
karate kick 10, 10, 10
one-leg squat 5, 5, 5
rear lunge 10, 10
plyometric jump 10
lunge jump 10
knee-tuck jump 10
bounds 20
hops 20

Friday
WORKOUT 3: PULL
pull-up 10, 10, 5, 5, 5
hanging knee raise 10, 10, 10
straight-arm pull 20, 20, 20
underhand pull-up 5, 5, 5
wide-grip pull-up 5, 5, 5
bend and reach 30
cobra stretch 5
extend and flex 20
forward bend 20
forward jump 10, 10, 10
windmill 20

Tuesday, Thursday, and Saturday
WORKOUT 4: RUN
The Long 12: on a track, run 6 laps, jogging the curves and sprinting the straightaways, going for the shortest sprint times on each of the 12 sprints

ROUTINE 8: PLYO

Plyometrics mix it up with concurrent training, as you run three miles but stop every 500 feet or so to do a burst of strength activity. You should be ready for plyometrics (able to do five clap push-ups, three full one-leg squats, and a 100-yard sprint) before trying this routine. Run three miles but stop every 500 feet or so to do a burst of strength activity. For the Run workout, use two markers, 2-by-1-inch rectangles cut from neon-bright heavy stock paper, a watch with a stopwatch, and a flat, grassy area. The markers let you visualize the distance, which doesn't have to be exact, so you can try for the best time on each sprint. Do this routine the second half of the third month to finish the three-month cycle.

Monday
WORKOUT 1: PUSH and WORKOUT 4: RUN
combine a 3-mile run with
push-up 30, 20
clap push-up 5, 5
dive bomb 10, 10
jump out 10, 10
plyometric jump out 5, 5
plyometric push-up 10, 10

Wednesday
WORKOUT 2: LIFT and WORKOUT 4: RUN
combine a 3-mile run with
deep squat 20, 20
contact squat 20, 20
forward lunge 10, 10
plyometric jump 10, 10
zig-zag jump 10
sideways jump 10, 10
pike jump 10

Friday
WORKOUT 3: PULL and WORKOUT 4: RUN
combine a 3-mile run with
pull-up 10, 10, 5, 5, 5, 5
hanging knee raise 10, 10
straight-arm pull 10, 10
wide-grip pull-up 5, 5

Tuesday, Thursday, and Saturday
WORKOUT 4: RUN
jog a mile, then, using markers, The Short 12:
sprint about 40 yards (36 meters) 12 times,
walking back to the starting marker after each
sprint, then jog a mile

ROUTINE 9: SPRINTER

This zeroes in on lower body strength and sprint capacity. Do as an alternate routine for the third month.

Monday
WORKOUT 4: RUN
interval training: The 1-to-5:
if "5" is your fastest 1-minute sustainable
sprint, run 1st minute at a "1," 2nd at a "2," 3rd
at a "3," 4th at a "4," and 5th minute at a "5,"
repeat 4 times for a 20-minute workout

Wednesday
WORKOUT 4: RUN
jog a mile, The Short 12: sprint 35 meters or
38 yards 12 times, allowing 10 seconds rest
between each sprint, then jog a mile

Thursday
WORKOUT 4: RUN
speed drill: foot turnovers 20, 20, 20
speed drill: laterals 20, 20, 20
speed drill: verticals 20, 20, 20
on a track, run 4 laps, walking the curves
but sprinting the straightaways, going for
best sprint times

Saturday
WORKOUT 4: RUN
the suicide drill: on a field, start at goal line,
sprint to nearest line, touch it with hand,
sprint back to goal, repeat for each line on
field, going for best overall time

Tuesday and Friday
WORKOUT 1: PUSH, WORKOUT 2: LIFT,
WORKOUT 3: PULL, and WORKOUT 4:
RUN
run approximately 1½ miles
push-up 30, 20, 20
plyometric jump out 5, 5, 5
plyometric push-up 10, 10
deep squat 20, 20, 20
forward lunge 10, 10, 10
one-leg squat 5, 5, 5
pull-up 10, 10, 5
bounds 20, 20, 20
hops 20, 20, 20
jog approximately 1½ miles

ROUTINE 10: JUMP START

Okay, so you have a busy life and there's no time for working out, no matter how you rearrange your schedule. Try this for a month. As promised, all it asks is 20 minutes, three days a week of strength exercise – plus whatever you're doing for cardio.

Monday and every other Friday
WORKOUT 1: PUSH
push-up 10, 10, 10
air boxing 1 minute
dive bomb 3, 2
jump out 5, 5
triceps push-up 5, 5
WORKOUT 2: LIFT
deep squat 20, 20
contact squat 20
forward lunge 10, 10
karate kick 10
plyometric jump (or gentle jump) 10

Wednesday and every other Friday
WORKOUT 3: PULL
pull-up 3, 2 (or straight-arm pulls if a pull-up is too hard)
hanging knee raise 8, 7
cobra stretch 5
forward bend 10

Every day
WORKOUT 4: RUN
walk briskly, jog, or interval train at least 20 minutes,
separately or combined with a workout above

Now it's time to turn to the other side of the body improvement equation, how you eat.

Section 3

THE SEVEN STEPS OF NUTRITION

Your body can thrive on many kinds of food, but eating what is better for you can make you leaner, healthier, and filled with energy. New research is pointing the way to a completely new way of eating, based on whole foods derived from plants. Meals prepared this way cost less, are easier to prepare, and, best of all, are delicious. Contrast this with the average American's eating habits, which can leave you tired, prone to a host of health problems – and, all too frequently, hungry. A delicious new way of eating, supported by an abundance of scientific evidence, can bolster your health, provide high-quality, slow-burning stream of energy, and give you a new and longer life.

Our understanding of what constitutes good nutrition is changing profoundly. Current research gives new urgency to the need to reduce overall caloric intake, especially by cutting down on more processed forms of food, while caloric intake, not fat, is being revealed to be the primary culprit causing unwanted weight gain. New findings highlight the benefits of certain essential forms of fat, which are being found to add flavor without adding health risks, keep you sated longer, and make lower-calorie eating sustainable over a lifetime. Other foods, especially in overly processed forms, are being more clearly linked to various diseases. Even as research continues to uncover a growing number of health risks associated with eating animal-based and highly processed food, on the other side of the equation, it is also finding new and unexpected health benefits in consuming whole foods derived from plants.

These findings are guiding us to a new and substantially healthier cuisine. The earlier trickle of studies about the benefits of eating vegetables has grown into a deluge of evidence demonstrating the positive effects of a cuisine largely, if not exclusively, based on minimally processed forms of beans, fruits, nuts, vegetables, and whole grains. These foods are nutrient dense without being calorie dense, which means you can eat your fill even as you take in fewer calories, and they abound in taste and flavor. As the recipes of the next section will show, healthful eating need not mean going hungry or giving up an enjoyable food life, it means fresh, varied, and wholesome meals.

Few things are more personal than how you eat; it's understandable if you resist the prospect of change. All of us, exercisers especially, cling to our nutritional beliefs. Even if you are sure you follow perfect eating habits, look at the information here with an open mind. It's based on research findings that may surprise you. The seemingly minor difference between whole grains and refined starches, for example, can make you healthier or sicker, while low-fat diets can actually make blood sugar problems worse and can even increase obesity. Not only are fruit and vegetables good for you, they also come with a potent array of irreplaceable plant-derived compounds, or phytonutrients, with measurable benefits that are just beginning to be discovered. Meanwhile, the potato, by far the most popular vegetable, is also the only one you should probably cut back on. And, well-funded milk advertisements aside, not only are dairy foods unnecessary, they may in fact be promoting prostate cancer in men and ovarian cancer in women, for whom dairy intake actually associates with *increased* bone fractures.

The approach this evidence suggests is simple: reap the benefits of living a healthier and longer life by adapting, to as great an extent as you can, to a whole-food cuisine based on food derived from plants in minimally processed form. This move will reinforce the positive exercise changes you're making with equally positive nutritional improvements that can make a substantial difference in your health over your lifetime. We'll look at this new way of eating as a process of seven simple steps:

Step 1: Drink Mainly Water

Step 2: Whole Grain Makes a Whole Lot of Difference

Step 3: It's Not the Fat, It's the Calories

Step 4: Not Nonfat, But Right Fat

Step 5: Eat Plenty of Vegetables and Fruits

Step 6: Get Your Protein from Plants

Step 7: Use Supplements Wisely

To persuade you to change the way you eat, let's look more closely at this seven-step path, and at the research behind it.

Step 1: Drink Mainly Water

One of the first and best ways to begin changing your diet for the better is to replace most, if not all, of your beverages with water. Cold, clear, and refreshing, water makes up 50 percent of your body mass and 75 percent of your muscle mass. With zero calories, water tips the caloric balance in your favor, filling you up without fattening you up. Replace your other beverages with water, most or even all of the time. Replace soft drinks, milk, and even fruit juices with water, make it your beverage of choice, and you'll cut your energy intake by hundreds of calories a day.

The use of bottled water, which is often merely treated municipal tap water, continues to rise, resulting in "quality incidents,"[213] – as well as billions of empty plastic water bottles.[214] Though tap water is normally safe, it should be checked for purity because old pipes or polluted reservoirs can contaminate tap water with lead, mercury, and dozens of other contaminants. Some of these can stay in your body once ingested, or bioaccumulate, to eventually threaten your health. Finding out if your tap water is clean is a worthwhile and straightforward process. First, contact your city for a free report on local water quality. Then, use a state-licensed water testing service to verify that the water coming out of your faucet is clean. These steps will save you the trouble and expense of lugging bottled water home from the grocery store each week.

Liquid calories don't help you stay thin. Soft drinks and fruit juices quickly spike your bloodstream with a large dose of calories, and calories, as we will see, are what make you fat. Fruit juices do have nutrients, making them marginally better than soft drinks, which contain as much as seven teaspoons of sugar in a single serving. But your body absorbs virtually any form of liquid calories all too easily. For example, after finishing a run on a hot summer day, I was able to very unscientifically guzzle down half a 64-fluid-ounce bottle of Naked Juice Mighty

THE DEPARTMENT OF DEBUNKING
SPORTS DRINKS

Regardless of what the sports drink industry says, the best exercise beverage is water. Sports drinks cost Americans over $5.1 billion in 2013 alone, but they only deliver nutrients already present in a well-balanced diet, along with excess calories. Some sports drinks are as much as 40 percent sugar, so they actually hurt exercise performance as the sugar onslaught diverts fluid away from your muscles and into your digestive tract. The high-quality, fiber-rich foods this book advocates digest slowly, so their nutrients will fuel you even through long workouts. These foods also contain plenty of the ions that sports drink manufacturers worry so much about you losing through exercise. The next time you're thirsty, reach for water instead.

Mango All Natural 100% Juice Smoothie With No Sugar Added, ingesting 600 calories – almost a quarter of my daily intake – in 23 seconds. Whether from corn syrup, sugar cane, or fruit juice, liquid forms of sugar are quickly absorbed into your bloodstream, making your blood sugar surge, then drop, leaving you tired and in need of more calories all too soon. By drinking water, you shift the source of your calories to solid food, which digests more slowly. Don't worry, we'll be adding plenty of the delicious foods to your diet to make up for the loss of your favorite beverages. Making water your primary beverage is one way this diet slows the rate at which the food you eat gets converted to energy from a quick flash to a slow burn. Such a shift is perhaps the primary way this nutritional approach can improve your health.

Water also has a modest but measurable thermogenic (metabolism-raising) effect, with half a liter (17 ounces) reported to raise energy expenditure by 24 percent over the course of an hour after ingestion,[215] and increased fluid intake may associate with improved memory and attention, at least for 7-to-9-year-old children.[216] So how much water should you drink?

Well, it's hard to drink too much water. Our bodies can handle about 10 liters a day. Beyond that amount, the concentration of vital minerals, such as salt, slowly begins to get diluted. To dilute your ion concentration to a life-threatening level, you would have to drink some 20 liters in a single day. So how much water should you drink? A recent review could not find any scientific evidence in support of the "seemingly ubiquitous admonition" to drink eight 8-ounce glasses of water a day, or 1.9 liters,[217] yet a daily water intake of a 3.7 liters (0.9 gallons) for adult men and 2.7 liters (0.7 gallons) for adult women has been cited as being likely to meet the needs of a vast majority of people, although heat or strenuous exercise greatly increase your water need.[218] It is difficult though not impossible to drink too much water, particularly in the midst of very prolonged exercise, such as during marathons, when overzealous water drinking without the means to urinate has resulted in overly dilute concentrations of salt or other minerals, a condition called hyponatremia.[219] Death by drinking water is very rare but has occurred, as noted in a morbidly fascinating *Scientific American* article, which described these unexpected deaths: club-goers under the influence of ecstasy who drank large amounts of water while trying to rehydrate after a night of dancing and sweating; a 21-year-old man who died during fraternity hazing after being forced to drink excessive amounts of water between rounds of push-ups in a cold basement; and a 28-year-old woman who died after consuming some one-and-a-half gallons of water in three hours while refraining from urinating in order to win a very ill-advised radio contest, "Hold Your Wee for a Wii."[220]

With its modest thermogenic effect and complete absence of calories, perhaps the best advice is to drink your fill of water before, during, and after exercise, unless you're experimenting with mind-altering drugs, undergoing hazing, or participating in contests that limit access to a bathroom.

Step 2: Whole Grain Makes a Whole Lot of Difference

With its rich colors and complex, nutty flavors, whole grain is an important part of a healthy diet. Its flavorful and nutrient-rich outer coating adds taste and slows digestion, while refined grain, such as white rice, white bread, and regular pasta, overwhelm you with sugar much like soft drinks or fruit juices do, providing too many calories too soon. The crucial distinction between slow-digesting whole grain and fast-digesting refined grain has been lost in the hype that "all" carbohydrates are bad.

Not all carbohydrates are bad. From a dietary point of view, what seems to matter most for a carbohydrate, whether it's a grain, fruit, or vegetable, is how much it has been refined. While many fruits and vegetables make it to our plates largely intact, much of the grain most of us eat is refined: cracked, milled, or pulverized, its rough outer hull thrown away, along with the bulk of its nutrients. As whole wheat flour is refined into white flour, for example, it loses more than 20 different nutrients, including 25 percent of its protein, 70 percent of its iron, 78 percent of its fiber, and 95 percent of its vitamin E, resulting in a fast-digesting flour so poor in nutrients that manufacturers are legally required to artificially enrich it with vitamins.[222] Refined grains like white bread, white rice, and white pasta begin dissolving into their component sugars almost as soon as they are eaten.

THE DEPARTMENT OF DEBUNKING
LOW-CARB DIETS

By lumping all carbohydrates together as "bad," the low-carbohydrate diets have become very popular, but they neglect your body's preferred energy source. To replace the shunned carbs, proteins, usually from animal products, come with saturated fat and cholesterol that clog your blood vessels. Worse, carbohydrate deprivation can cause ketosis, a kind of blood poisoning whose hallmarks are fruity breath, headaches, nausea, and cramps, all of which signal your kidneys' struggle to manage your blood's rising acid levels. Even if you can manage to exercise in such a state, the lactic acid naturally produced by movement only adds to the burden on your overworked kidneys. Long-term carbohydrate restriction could have some serious consequences that include heart arrhythmia, kidney damage, increased cancer risk, osteoporosis, and even sudden death.[221] Instead of struggling to exercise in a ketotic state, consider cutting back on processed carbohydrates, and include more forms of whole carbohydrates like fruits, vegetables, and whole grains in your diet.

Well before such grain arrives in the intestine, its starchy flour has dissolved into glucose, a sugar. The resulting flood of sugar into your bloodstream triggers a chain of events that by now should sound familiar: the abundance of sugar triggers a flood of insulin, which hurries the sugar into your cells, and later instigates a blood sugar crash, making you feel tired and hungry again.

It's no coincidence this sounds like a description of diabetes. With repeated bouts of high blood sugar, your cells become resistant to insulin, the hormone that helps your cells access food sugar from the bloodstream, and higher amounts of insulin are needed to process the sugar. Your pancreas has to work harder and harder to secrete enough insulin to keep up. Eventually it burns out, and adult-onset diabetes results.[223, 224] This problem is compounded by faulty nutritional advice, including our own country's "food pyramid," in which refined grains like bread, pasta, and rice remain mainstays. Even in its recently revised form, the food pyramid still recommends that you consume half of your grain in refined form, despite the link between refined grain intake and adult-onset diabetes.[225] Following this faulty advice, many people load up on highly processed forms of grain like cornflakes, rice cakes, and white bread, not realizing these foods enter the bloodstream as sugar even faster than sugar itself.[226] The combination of poor advice and broadening availability of convenience foods, which are normally high in refined grain, is thought to be one reason why adult-onset diabetes has become epidemic.[227]

Instead of avoiding all carbohydrates, try to eat less refined grain and more whole grain. Brown rice, old-fashioned oats, whole grain bread, and delicious whole grains like amaranth, buckwheat, kasha, millet, quinoa, rye, and wild rice now appear in most well-stocked grocery stores. Amaranth has a nutty cereal-like flavor, and, like quinoa, it's packed with protein, as well as healthful forms of carbohydrate. Coarse breads like rye and pumpernickel (a sourdough rye) offer rich, substantial flavors. Wheat comes in an even less refined, therefore healthier, whole form as wheat berries, just as oats are available in their whole form as oat groats. As grocery stores begin to carry more whole grains, it will become easier to put them on the menu. If you do buy processed food, read the label. If it doesn't specifically say "whole" before the name of the grain, then it is probably the kind of fast-digesting refined grain you might be better off avoiding. Whole grains or flours can be boiled, sauteed, steamed, toasted, and mixed into doughs, stews, or pilafs. The longer cooking time they require, which might explain the virtual disappearance of whole grains off the fast-paced American menu of the last century, is offset by their better nutrients, health, and taste.

Whole grains also help keep you lean. Because they are harder to digest, they deliver their energy slowly over a longer period of time, like a time-release capsule, letting you go longer before your blood sugar level drops and triggers hunger. Because they deliver their calories more slowly, your body has more of a chance to use them for movement instead of storing them as fat. Keeping you satisfied longer, they let you take in fewer calories over a 24-hour period. Far from being carbohydrates to avoid, whole grains are a slow-burning, nutrient-rich, and lower-calorie source of energy to power you through the day.

So how much whole grain should you eat? Generally, one serving with each meal is plenty. A serving is a portion of food about the size of your closed fist. To introduce you to whole grains, the recipes in the next section start off with a breakfast rich in multiple forms of whole grain that doesn't require any cooking, and go on to include in subsequent dishes whole grain in all its forms.

Step 3: It's Not the Fat, It's the Calories

While the saying "a calorie is a calorie" is not quite true — the body captures energy from dietary fat more efficiently than from carbohydrate,[228] and diets emphasizing low fat intake do, at least initially, result in more body fat loss than those using normal fat intake[229,230] — over a lifetime, the primary way you get thin is by habitually consuming fewer calories than you burn.[231] The problem with going on a "diet" is that they don't work for more than a short time. Sooner or later, you go off the diet. Researchers investigating the high long-term failure rate of low-fat diets have found that the proportion of dietary fat in a diet poorly predicts its success over the course of a year or more, and note how in America, even though dietary fat intake has substantially declined, obesity has significantly increased.[232] You need a way to bring calorie intake under control without feeling like you have to starve yourself.

How many calories you need depends on who you are and how much physical activity you do: active females on average need about 2,000 calories a day, and active males need about 3,000,[233] although these numbers vary depending on your size, age, amount of daily exercise (which directly burns calories), and amount of muscle tissue (which indirectly burns calories). However, if you're living in an industrialized society, it's a safe bet that you are taking in more calories than you need. There is no simpler way to live better, to live longer — really, to be happier — than to cut the number of calories you consume.

Then harness the power of exercise to burn calories. The effectiveness of this two-pronged strategy of cutting calories *and* exercising is underscored by studies showing how strongly the lack of it contributes to obesity. Young obese women, for example, have been shown to continue to gain more weight than their normal-weight peers on *fewer* calories due to their lower level of physical activity.[235] Just as exercise raises metabolism by building muscle, inactivity lowers metabolism because muscle that is not used will waste away, or atrophy. Your body only builds muscle if it needs to. If you exercise, in whatever way you can manage, you will lose weight over time by increasing the energy you burn each day.

In addition to emphasizing exercise, to lose body fat in a culture where food is all too available, it might be helpful also to learn to eat defensively.

THE DEPARTMENT OF DEBUNKING
FAT-FREE FOODS

Supporters of the idea that eating fat makes you fat often cite the fact that a gram of fat yields nine calories while a gram of protein or carbohydrates yields only four. Even the United States Department of Agriculture was still recommending avoiding all fats until 2005, when it finally retired the Food Pyramid under a cloud of controversy. Fat has the advantage of triggering your body's satiety mechanism to give you that full feeling. Deliberately adding a limited amount of fat, as one study did by adding almonds to a meal, actually results in fewer calories being consumed overall.[234] Fat also slows digestion, delaying the return of hunger. Without it, blood sugar surges higher and plunges lower, leaving you feeling tired and hungry, so you eat again. This is especially a problem for overweight, obese, and diabetic people, who experience wider swings in blood sugar in response to sugary and starchy food. If they try to follow a nonfat diet, a vicious circle emerges: weight gain, a redoubled effort to stick to nonfat foods, and more hunger. Often the weight gain leads to further nonfat dieting, but hunger always wins in the end, and the diet fails. When it does, the ensuing caloric deluge is especially disastrous: primed by famine, the dieter's body efficiently sequesters every extra calorie to store it away as fat.

- *Practice the fine art of portion control.* Pay attention to how much you put on your plate or in your bowl, since most of us tend to keep eating until the dish is clean. Take a cue from nouvelle cuisine restaurants and make smaller portions look bigger by switching to smaller dishes. You will often find that a smaller portion eaten more slowly can be just as filling as a larger but hurried meal.

- *If you are hungry, take your time and enjoy the food.* It takes time for your body to tell you that you're full, so the faster you eat, the more calories you'll consume before you get the signal that you've had enough. Too frequently, we allow ourselves only a short time to eat, but your satiation mechanism doesn't move at a modern pace. Try to slow down and enjoy your meals, and you will feel sated before you take in too much. It's worthwhile to take the time you need to eat food slowly so that you feel full.

- *Get thrown out of the clean plate club.* Don't feel like you have to finish everything in front of you. It's hard to estimate exactly how much food you actually need when you serve yourself a portion. As you near the end of a meal, don't feel guilty for not finishing all of it. Leaving an unfinished plate is better than carrying extra weight.

- *When you're done, you're done.* When finished eating, brush your teeth. Help wash the dishes. Leave the eating room. These small gestures show yourself that you've finished.

- *Ride the wave.* If you're trying to lose weight, you do have to run a caloric deficit, and that does mean there will be times when you feel hungry as you get used to eating less. If hunger hits, don't rush to satisfy the urge. Wait. The wave of hunger will crest and subside.

- *Eat only for sustenance.* Eat for hunger, not for social or emotional reasons. In our workplaces, our homes, and our social events, we're constantly being offered food. Instead of eating just out of politeness or tradition, think about the food available to you. Do you need to eat it now? Are you truly hungry, or are you eating just for social reasons? While there are worse ways to handle stress than eating food, be wary of substituting food for better ways of dealing with adversity. Maybe a good talk with a family member, a phone call, or a visit with a friend over coffee is a better way than eating food for dealing with emotional distress.

- *Eat on your own time.* Follow an eating pattern that makes sense for you. Except for the desirability of ingesting protein soon after strength exercise if you wish to promote muscle growth,[236] meal timing does not seem to significantly influence calorie intake or perceived hunger,[237] although eating less than three times a day may slow your metabolism and can make it hard to control your appetite,[238] and reduced sleep does appear to be a risk factor for weight gain.[239] Following a consistent schedule that allows for sufficient exercise, the consumption of at least three meals a day at regular times,[240] and all the sleep you need may require a little simplifying of your schedule, but will be more likely to keep you feeling satisfied and help you avoid unwanted weight gain.

Step 4: Not Nonfat, but Right Fat

Instead of trying to omit all fat, distinguish the good from the bad. You can use the good forms of fat, which derive from plant-based sources, to feel more satisfied on less food, make your meals taste better, and keep your calorie intake under control. Instead of getting stuck on a diet of bland, quick-digesting, nonfat foods, use a small amount of fat in its healthy forms to make your meals tasty, filling, and good for you: a little bit of the right kind of fat can help you get thin.

Fat in moderation is useful. It cushions body organs like your eyes and kidneys, insulates you, is used to build cellular membranes and nerve sheathing, serves as a concentrated source of energy, and triggers satiety. Its smooth, buttery taste intensifies other flavors in foods. Vitamins A, D, E, and K dissolve only in fat, so you'll need it to absorb these potent antioxidants into your body. The fat in foods also slows the process of stomach emptying, prolonging digestion and delaying the return of hunger.

While all forms of fat share this desirable effect of slowing the release of food energy into your body, not all forms of it are good for you. Fat in solid form is called saturated fat because each molecule is chemically saturated with hydrogen, that is, each of its carbon atoms forms the maximum possible number of bonds to hydrogen atoms instead of forming additional bonds to other carbon atoms. This kind of fat stays solid at room temperature, making it easy to identify. Much of the fat in dairy products (including butter), meat, and other animal-based food is saturated. Your blood transports saturated fat in fragile packets that break along their course through the blood vessels, strewing their contents along the vessel walls. Over time, diets high in saturated fat cause heart disease and other medical problems (like high blood pressure, peripheral vascular disease, and strokes), which develop as the blood vessels throughout the body narrow and eventually completely clog with solidified fat.[241] The saturated fat in meat and dairy foods is accompanied by a form of cholesterol that promotes and accelerates the growth of solid fat deposits along blood vessel walls. Vascular damage begins early in life: autopsies of 760 young Americans who had died from external (non-medical) causes found 2 percent of teenagers and 20 percent of 30-to-35-year-olds already carried advanced atherosclerotic plaque in their major blood vessels.[242]

The other "bad" kind of fat, hydrogenated fat, also known as "trans fat," is entirely man-made. Hydrogenation simply means adding hydrogen to the fat on a molecular level, so that more of its carbon atoms bind with hydrogen, making it more closely resemble saturated fat. Manufacturers hydrogenate plant-derived fats like soybean, corn, palm, and other oils to extend their shelf life so they won't spoil during storage in warehouses or on grocery shelves. Although it is beginning to be phased out, hydrogenated fat can still be found in hydrogenated soybean oil (found in margarine), inexpensive peanut butter, snacks, and many convenience foods, as well as in vegetable shortening, often used in pastries and restaurant cooking.

Unfortunately, hydrogenating fat has consequences. In the body, it aggressively displaces healthier forms of fat to clog vessels even more tenaciously than saturated fat. Hydrogenated fat consumption is associated with blood vessel damage, even after accounting for multiple other factors, including age, weight, exercise, smoking, alcohol consumption, and fat intake.[243] You can avoid hydrogenated fat the same way you can avoid most saturated fat, by choosing foods made from largely unprocessed forms of beans, fruits, nuts, vegetables, and whole grains. Before you buy a processed food like bread or breakfast cereal, read the label. If the ingredients include hydrogenated fat or vegetable shortening, don't buy it. If you eat out frequently, ask for foods low in saturated fat and free of trans fat.

Fat that comes from plants, on the other hand, tends to take liquid form – oil – at room temperature. These plant-sourced fats are mostly "unsaturated" because more of their carbon atoms are bound to each other instead of to hydrogen. Provided it has not been subjected to hydrogenation, the fat in canola, flaxseed, olive, peanut, safflower oil, and nuts is predominantly unsaturated. Canola oil, made from rapeseed, has among all the oils the lowest percent of saturated fat, only 6 percent. Each kind of plant oil has its own flavor and combination of nutrients and is high in unsaturated fat. A glaring exception is the currently fashionable coconut. Coconut oil is unusual because of its high saturated fat content: some 89 percent of the fat in coconut oil is saturated, and it carries a whopping 11.7-gram amount of saturated fat – 58 percent of a day's entire recommended amount – in a single tablespoon.

Unsaturated fat works on your blood vessels like a drain opener, helping scrub away the deposits left by saturated fat.[244] One kind of unsaturated fat, called omega-3, is an essential nutrient that cannot be manufactured by your body on its own, but rather must be included in food. Omega-3 fat forms an important component in cell membranes, especially for brain and sperm cells, and is thought to help reduce the risk of blood clotting and heart arrhythmia.[245] It may even mitigate the risk of autoimmune disorders like eczema, lupus, and rheumatoid arthritis.[246] Many kinds of plant-derived fats are abundant in omega-3 fat, especially canola oil, flaxseed, and walnuts.

Fat carries a lot of energy, so you don't need very much of it. A few tablespoons of oil a day or the equivalent amount in nuts should give you all the essential fat you need. Plant-derived fats in forms like olive oil or canola oil as well as the fat in nuts, seeds, and plant-based milks are all higher in healthier unsaturated fats and lower in saturated fat. Canola oil, freshly ground flaxseed, and walnuts are especially high in the essential omega-3 form of unsaturated fat.

Step 5: Eat Plenty of Vegetables and Fruits

There's little doubt that fruits and vegetables are good for you. A wealth of studies investigating the diverse benefits of fruits and vegetables and their nutrients suggest that medical science validates the truth of your mother's sage advice: eat lots of fruits and vegetables. In addition to vitamins and minerals, plants contain literally thousands of other compounds that boost your health and prevent disease in a remarkable variety of ways, from lowering blood pressure to reducing age-related memory loss. For example, investigators at the University of Oxford studied 10,000 people over a 17-year period and found that a vegetarian diet is associated with reduced risk of colorectal cancer, and note that substances in fruits and vegetables may inhibit the triggering of cancerous cell growth. They also found that the bile acid secreted in response to the fat of red meat encourages tumor growth.[247] Another study shows that men who eat three daily servings of cruciferous vegetables are 41 percent less likely to develop prostate cancer.[248] (Cruciferous vegetables include beet greens, broccoli, Brussels sprouts, cabbage, cauliflower, collard greens, kale, mustard greens, radishes, and Swiss chard, among others.) Sage and also lemon balm improve memory in people with Alzheimer's and dementia.[249] Vegetable protein reduces the risk of gall bladder disease[250] and a study of 118,000 men and women has found that eating as few as three servings of fruit a day is associated with a 36 percent reduction percent in the risk of macular degeneration, an age-related cause of blindness with few effective treatment options.[251]

High in bulk but low in calories, vegetables and fruits let you fill up without getting fat. In addition to health-boosting phytonutrients, fruits and vegetables, like whole grains and "good" forms of fat, provide a high-quality, slow-burning source of energy. Fruits and vegetables are high in cellulose, an indigestible form of fiber, which does not itself turn into calories but slows the digestion of the portion of fruit or vegetable that does. That means your body converts the digestible components of fruits and vegetables into energy slowly so your blood sugar stays more even, you stay sated longer, and can go longer before getting hungry.

So foods from the plant kingdom can provide a foundation for lifelong, life-sustaining eating. The advice to load up on minimally processed forms of vegetables and fruits, however, comes with three interesting caveats concerning fruit juice, potatoes, and tomatoes.

First, as mentioned before (page 69), fruit juices pack an enormous number of calories into a quickly digestible liquid. You really should think of fruit juice, no matter how assertively the packaging mentions the inclusion of pulp or natural ingredients, as a form of processed food that is best consumed only parsimoniously. "Processing" means any procedure that changes food from its natural form to the form it appears in just before you eat it. Peeling a banana is a form of food processing, as is extruding the pulp of a banana into a mixture of refined flour, sorbitol, cornstarch, partially hydrogenated soybean oil, and maltodextrin, to list the first five ingredients in a popular banana cake mix. Nobody is suggesting you need to start eating banana peels, but excessive food processing seems to generally lead to degraded nutritional quality and tends to introduce man-made ingredients that often seem to become implicated, sooner or later, in causing some kind of biological harm. It is not all food processing that current research cautions against, just excessive processing, such as augmenting water to produce sugary sports drinks, stripping grain of its hull, hydrogenating fat, or mingling fruits and vegetables with a stew of chemicals. One hundred percent pure fruit juice, marketed as a way to add fruit to your diet, is manufactured by stripping its peel and pulverizing its flesh to squeeze out a liquid packed with calories that can be absorbed very quickly. So the advice to load up on plenty of fruit and vegetables should not apply to fruit juices; no matter how aggressively the packaging tells you otherwise, think of fruit juice as a liquid form of fruit sugar – in other words, a processed treat that you might be better off enjoying sparingly.

Next, the potato, all too frequently the only vegetable Americans regularly eat, is also the only one you probably should cut back on. One problem with advocating completely vegetarian eating is that people often lose the meat from their diet but keep the potatoes. Like white bread, pancakes, and other low-quality carbohydrates, potatoes – whether baked or mashed, in latkes or in French fries – are packed with starch that floods your bloodstream with sugar all too quickly. If potatoes were just an occasional indulgence, this wouldn't be a problem, but the potato is the most popular American vegetable, often replacing or substituting for healthier vegetable alternatives. Step off of the potato merry-go-round – almost any other fruit or vegetable makes a better choice.

Finally, tomatoes, unlike virtually all other vegetables and fruits, become *more* nutritious during processing: pulverizing and cooking them in a little bit of oil frees up cancer-preventing[252,253] antioxidants called lycopenes that are bound up in the tomato's cell walls, making tomatoes an odd exception to the idea that processing degrades food. While shucking the hull and throwing away the endosperm reduces the nutrient quality and deleteriously speeds up the digestibility of grain, and extracting juice from fruit results in beverages with delicious taste but an industrial-strength amount of calories, subjecting tomatoes to mechanical processes like dicing, pulverizing, or cooking them into paste actually improves their nutritional value by prying lycopenes out, increasing their bioavailability,[254] as does cooking them in a small amount of oil.[255]

Experts recommend you eat at least five servings of vegetables and fruits each day. To get their full benefit, go for variety and try new colors, shapes, and textures. Different colors signal the presence of different phytonutrients, with deeper, richer colors generally signifying their greater abundance. The plant kingdom offers us a feast of color and taste: the sweet, tangy yellows and oranges of the citrus family; the oranges, reds, and purples of tomatoes, peppers, radishes, and beets; the savory richness of garlic and onions; and the deep iron-rich greens of cabbage, collard greens, kale, and spinach. As vegetarianism becomes more popular, produce sections are becoming livelier and more diverse, making it easier to find appealing vegetables and fruits. To avoid degrading the content or quality of phytonutrients, try to obtain most of your vegetables or fruits in raw or home-cooked form. You should look for every opportunity to add them. Include them as a side dish for any meal, even breakfast. It's worthwhile to make the effort to consume fresh fruits and vegetables, and once you regularly do so for a while, the habit will stick. Sweet jumbo mixed red, gold and purple raisins compliment good old-fashioned apples, bananas, and citrus. Seasons bring fresh food closer, with spring's dandelion greens, radishes, rhubarb, and wild onions, summer's succession of strawberries, raspberries, gooseberries, and blueberries, late summer's green beans and zucchini, and fall's corn, plums, grapes, squash, walnuts, and chestnuts. You can cut up and combine vegetables that refrigerate well and stay fresh all week long, like baby broccoli, collard greens, kale, purple cabbage, spinach, Swiss chard, and watercress. Other vegetables, like carrots, celery root, golden beets, (peeled) jicama, fennel, kohlrabi, radishes, sweet potatoes, and turnips slice easily in a food processor to make a colorful salad. Experiment with a variety of raw and home-cooked vegetable and fruit dishes. Instead of adding a sugary dressing, try the subtler flavors of fresh herbs like basil, cilantro, dill, mint, parsley, sage, scallions, or tarragon. By making leaves and roots a primary food, seeking out variety, welcoming traditional and new forms of minimally processed foods, and finding local seasonal produce, fruits and vegetables can form the foundation of a satisfying cuisine that will sustain you for life.

Step 6: Get Your Protein from Plants

Many of us get most of our protein from meat and dairy, which also come with a host of health, hygiene, and environmental problems. You can switch to a variety of plant-based food – beans, fruits, nuts, vegetables, and whole grains – and still get protein enough. At the same time, you'll be consuming less saturated fat, more fiber, no cholesterol, and far fewer calories. You'll also be opening up your food world to new and varied colors, textures, and tastes. Plant-based eating over a lifetime profoundly reduces the financial and ecological costs of living, and diets comprised exclusively of such foods, called vegan (usually pronounced "VEE-gun"), relate, in a growing body of research, to a leaner, healthier, better, and longer life. Changing to a completely vegan diet is one of the smartest things you can do to make a brighter future for you and for our planet.

Nitrogen balance studies, which measure protein's absorption and release in the body, have resulted in a recommended daily allowance, or RDA, of 0.38 grams of protein for each pound of body weight (or 0.8 grams of protein per kilogram),[256] which works out to be 63 grams of protein a day for a 175-pound person. The 0.38-gram-protein-per-pound-bodyweight recommendation is thought to be enough to stave off muscle loss and meet the protein needs of more than 97 percent of the population,[257] excluding women more than three months pregnant (0.4 grams), nursing mothers (0.5 grams) – and strength-training athletes seeking bigger muscles (0.7 grams). Americans already typically consume some 150 percent of the recommended protein amount every day,[258] with dispiriting results, as a quick look around a shopping mall or crowded train station may confirm. Nonetheless, if you are trying to increase your muscle mass, there is definitely evidence that recommends getting a higher protein intake above the RDA minimum. Analysis of some 22 randomized trials showed that among 680 total subjects, protein supplementation increased muscle mass and strength,[259] that protein supplementation was not just helpful but required to stimulate muscle gain for frail elderly people doing strength training,[260] and an intriguing study even noted that higher dietary protein intake by itself largely predicted greater hamstring strength in blue-collar workers,[261] because protein consumption increases muscle protein synthesis.[262]

Yet over the long term, higher protein intake also has its costs, detailed in the sidebar on the right, especially with regard to disease processes, which, once started, can derail a life. Consumption of vegetable protein, as distinct from animal protein, relates to lower blood pressure,[278] lower levels of cholesterol,[279] better cardiovascular health,[280] lower risk of diabetes,[281] better functioning among arthritis sufferers,[282] and longer life.[283] So if you're doing strength training and trying to gain muscle, you might consider adding some plant protein, as directed in Recipe #3, Energizer Oat Breakfast (page 93). Otherwise, you might be better off emphasizing the long term over the short term, and just follow the RDA recommended amount of 0.38 grams protein per pound of body weight per day.

Plants do contain protein, if in modest amounts. Beans provide an average of 20 grams of protein in each serving, and there are about 12 grams of protein per serving in many kinds of whole grains: amaranth, brown rice, buckwheat, millet, oats, quinoa, rye, triticale, and whole wheat. While providing an average of 6 grams of protein per serving, nuts also deliver a diverse array of health-boosting phytonutrients like isoflavonoids,[284] polyphenols,[285] and phytosterols,[286] which have all been shown to promote cardiovascular health and prevent several types of cancer.[287] Vegetables, which you may think of as a carbohydrate source, also contain protein. Even the humble mushroom has 3 grams of protein and 25 percent of the United States RDA for fiber in a single serving, all for only 25 calories. Three meals made from beans, nuts, whole grains, fruits, and vegetables can handily yield more than the 63 grams of protein minimum needed every day by a 175-pound person.

Proteins are made from 20 amino acids and of these, nine are considered essential because your body can't synthesize them from other amino acids. Like the omega-3 form of unsaturated fat, these nine amino acids must be included in your food regularly. In the world of plant protein, soy is unique in containing a nearly complete amino acid profile, containing all nine of the essential amino acids, and having long been known to be as effective as beef for maintaining nitrogen balance.[288] The Food and Drug Administration has recognized that soy reduces risk of heart disease,[289] and that it may diminish arthritis,[290] cholesterol,[291] and prostate cancer risk as well.[292] Findings like these should be enough to sell you on soy, but what of any risks? Is there a downside to consuming soy?

THE DEPARTMENT OF DEBUNKING
HIGH-PROTEIN DIETS

High-protein diets like Atkins can help you lose weight initially, but they rely heavily on foods high in animal-based protein, which carries a dangerous load of saturated fat and cholesterol that primes your body for heart disease and other health problems down the road. These are drawbacks that overshadow a weight loss that might only be temporary. In one of the few studies looking beyond the short-term effects of the Atkins diet, researchers found that dieters following a high-protein calorie-restricted diet did lose weight over the first six months,[263] but, perhaps because the dietary regimen was unappetizing,[264] by 12 months they had gained the weight back, leaving them no better off than other dieters.[265] Atkins dieters not only regained the lost weight after a year, but continued to report cramps, headaches, and muscle weakness, which the researchers suggested might be at least partly related to the reduced intake of fruits, vegetables, and whole grain.[266] High-protein diets increase bone fracture risk[267] by removing calcium from the body,[268] hurt kidneys,[269, 270, 271] and can more than double your risk of kidney stones,[272, 273, 274, 275] an acutely painful event that happens to 12 percent of us over our lifetimes. Finally, chronic high protein intake associates with diabetes, obesity, and early death.[276, 277] Findings like these give further reason to consider obtaining your protein from plants.

Soy is also a phytoestrogen, which means that it's a plant nutrient that weakly mimics the human hormone estrogen. Since human estrogen inhibits muscle-building testosterone and may also trigger certain processes in breast cancer formation, it has been hypothesized that too much soy could increase breast cancer risk in women, and adversely affect testosterone levels in men (see "The Male Soy Scare" at left). A short-term study showed soy increasing breast cell proliferation, which suggested it might hasten breast cancer development as well,[293] but a later long-term study of 1,459 breast cancer patients has shown no link between soy intake and cancer survival.[294] These findings suggest that while you might not want to go overboard with soy you could include it in your diet in moderation along with a variety of other plant-sourced proteins.

Even plant-sourced foods that by themselves lack all the essential amino acids still yield a complete amino acid array when combined. Beans with brown rice, peas with corn, or lentils with whole grain bread are all combinations that contain sufficient amounts of the nine essential amino acids. You can see the pattern: beans paired with grains. Just by eating a variety of food, you can obtain all nine amino acids in one meal, even if you consume plant-based foods exclusively.[295] As a review published in the *American Journal of Clinical Nutrition* observed, "mixtures of plant proteins can serve as a complete and well-balanced source of amino acids for meeting human physiological requirements."[296]

Along with the research supporting the health benefits of plant-sourced food, evidence is also accumulating to link meat and dairy with health problems. Meat, especially from land animals, is not only high in saturated fat and cholesterol, but charred, grilled, or well-done meat is also loaded with heterocyclic amines, which are suspected to be carcinogenic, as suggested by a long-term study relating red meat consumption to a 40 percent increase in the risk of colon cancer.[297] Animal protein consumption also seems to increase the risk of non-Hodgkin lymphomas, with red meat consumption doubling the relative risk of these serious and difficult-to-treat cancers, and non-red meat consumption increasing the risk by 52 percent, according to a study published in the *Journal of the American Medical Association*.[298] The saturated fat and cholesterol that comes from meat impairs blood vessels function,[299] and has long been known to increase your risk of heart disease, high blood pressure, peripheral vascular disease, and stroke.[300]

Compounding the problem is the quality of much of today's farm-raised meat. Victims of the relentless logic of market forces, animals raised for meat usually live out short, miserable lives in cramped space, getting little or no physical activity, and being fed a diet of low-quality, rapidly digesting carbohydrate, because this treatment saves money,[301] even though it is also known to further raise the saturated fat level in their meat.[302,303]

This might explain why a large-scale study of some 38,000 people has shown that meat eaters are on average the most overweight people, and vegans the leanest.[304] The economic pressure to bring meat to the market at a reasonable price inevitably results in mass production, concentration, transport, and slaughter, which harm the animals involved in ways that also degrade the quality of the meat that their carcasses yield.[305,306] Then there is the "gross-out" factor in meat production: *Fast Food Nation: The Dark Side of the All-American Meal* has documented cramped warehouses reeking of ammonia, urine, and feces, where animals destined for slaughter live in crowded pens and eat food laced with antibiotics, steroids, and sedatives. Such practices occasionally result in public health problems, including incidental fecal contamination of meat destined for grocery store shelves, or well-publicized outbreaks of *E. coli* bacterial infections. The animals are also sometimes accidently or even purposely fed meal mixed with the ground-up remains of their own species, a ghoulish practice suspected of spreading "mad cow" disease, caused by biologically active proto-viruses called prions present in animal brain or spinal cord tissue.[307] Even aided by the macabre efficiency of such practices, the "factory farm" meat and dairy industry puts immense strain on the planet's limited capacity for producing food. Besides herbicides, pesticides, and other pollutants, 50 pounds of grain are needed to produce a single pound of beef. That means an acre of land can potentially support 50 times as many vegetarians as meat eaters. Removing meat from your diet therefore carries a triple benefit: it helps your health, reduces animal suffering, and eases the strain on an overpopulated planet.

The second major protein source for most Americans is dairy, most often in the form of milk. Along with protein, milk contains lactose – a sugar that, by some estimates, more than half of the world's population can't digest.[308] Because few of us can completely break down all of the lactose in a glass of milk, you may find that reducing the amount of milk you drink will make you less feel gassy even if lactose doesn't give you overt bloating, diarrhea, or nausea. Many of the proteins in milk are antigenic – they activate the immune system – and are thought to aggravate a variety of autoimmune disorders including asthma,[309] eczema,[310] and even arthritis.[311] The three daily glasses of low-fat milk recommended by the milk-industry-funded National Dairy Council put some 330 extra calories into your body every day, and filling those three glasses with whole milk would give you even more calories, not to mention more saturated fat than a dozen strips of bacon.

So why drink milk? "For the calcium, which builds strong bones," most people would say, echoing the National Dairy Council's popular "Got Milk?" campaign. But it is physical activity, not calcium, that makes strong bones. While the relationship between weight-bearing exercise and bone density is well-understood (page 14), the relationship between calcium consumption and bone density is, in the words of one meta-analysis, "very small, if any." The same analysis suggests that calcium intake has little or no effect on fracture prevention.[312] A long-term study of 60,689 women similarly has failed to show any significant relationship between dietary calcium and the risk of bone fractures.[313] While short-term calcium supplements provide a small increase in bone mass, over the long term, your body adapts to the high calcium intake and the net change in bone mass is minimal. The very readable *Eat, Drink, and Be Healthy: The Harvard Medical School Guide to Healthy Eating* cites a long-term study of Scandinavian male prisoners whose calcium intake was ultra-low at less than 500 milligrams of calcium per day. Despite this low level of dietary calcium, their bodies simply adapted to store and use it more efficiently.[314] It also cites still another long-term study on women and hip fractures that shows women in countries with lower per capita calcium consumption have *fewer* hip fractures. Women in countries with an average calcium intake of more than 1,000 milligrams per day actually suffer almost double the number of hip fractures as women in countries where per capita calcium intake is less than 1,000 milligrams per day.[315]

In contrast to the equivocal relationship between calcium and bone strength, plenty of studies show fairly clearly that people who exercise, whether soccer players,[316] joggers,[317] or just active people,[318] have stronger bones. The studies suggest that physical activity, not dairy intake, might be the primary factor associated with strong bones; besides, plant-based foods, particularly dark green leafy vegetables like kale, collard greens, turnip greens, Swiss chard, and broccoli, contain calcium enough to replace the loss incurred by abstaining from dairy.

Worse than allergies, bloating, extra calories, or lack of proven necessity, there is some real evidence that milk products carry health risks. An *American Journal of Clinical Nutrition* study has shown that men with higher dairy product intake are three times as likely to develop advanced prostate cancer and four times as likely to develop metastatic prostate cancer as men who consume dairy products in lower amounts;[319] while two separate meta-analyses conclude that dairy intake increases prostate cancer risk,[320, 321] and scientists suspect that dairy consumption may also be linked to ovarian cancer.[322] Evidence like this is behind recommendations to exclude dairy even from a vegetarian diet,[323] which adds to the evidence in favor of an exclusively plant-sourced diet.

As human activity continues to introduce poisons like herbicides, pesticides, and other toxins into the environment, some of these substances biodegrade, but some do not, and these find their way into the food supply.[324, 325] Each time an herbivore eats a contaminated plant, it retains approximately 10 percent of any toxin that was in the ingested plant, oxidizing or excreting the rest.[326] By eating a contaminated herbivore, a carnivore likewise permanently retains about 10 percent of whatever toxin was present in the herbivore. Repeated feedings on contaminated plants allow herbivores to accumulate, over their lifetimes, toxin levels far higher than that found in the plants they consume, and carnivores repeatedly consuming the meat or milk of contaminated herbivores likewise can accumulate toxins at higher levels still.[327, 328] In this way, toxins, once introduced into the environment, concentrate as they move up the food chain, with the highest levels found in the liver, kidneys, as well as fatty tissues such as the brain and spinal cord of any animal, including human, at the top.[329] While eating plants does not completely eliminate the risk of ingesting toxins, not consuming meat or dairy guarantees entry to the food chain at a lower level to substantially lower your exposure.

If you think you require meat and dairy in order to build strong muscle and bone, you might consider the work of researchers at St Louis's Washington University School of Medicine. They studied raw-food vegans (who eschew not only meat and dairy but also high-temperature cooking) by examining their bones with dual-energy x-ray absorptiometry, a technique that can be used to search for bone fractures. In all of the raw-food vegans (who had been following the diet for an average of 3.6 years), out of more than 3,700 bones (18 raw-food vegans each having about 206 bones apiece), not one bone had any evidence of a fracture. Additionally, the bones of raw-food vegans had other indications of better health. The raw-food vegans' bones had markedly more vitamin D, and lower levels of C-reactive protein and IGF-1, substances linked with heart disease, diabetes, and several types of cancer. The vegans also had a healthier body weight than the control group of traditional eaters, who were overweight.[330] Even children who grow up eating vegan enjoy good, even superior nutrition, provided they consume a variety of foods and take a multivitamin.[331]

Consider two dinners, one of plant-sourced food, the other, steak and potatoes:

THE DINNER MATCHUP: PLANT VS. ANIMAL

DINNER	DINNER SIZE	% US RDA OF PROTEIN	CALORIES	SATURATED FAT
minestrone (a 17-oz. bowl of minestrone, 3.6-oz whole grain crackers, a 7-oz. fresh salad with a scoop of peanut butter, and an apple)	35 oz.	63%	1,177	6 grams
steak and potatoes (an 8-oz. tenderloin steak with an 8-oz. baked potato, 2 pats of butter, a parsley sprig, and an 8-oz. glass of milk)	25 oz.	108%	1,277	68 grams

This example also illustrates yet another benefit of going vegan: you can eat more, but less. Even though the vegan dinner, comprised of generous-sized servings of Minestrone (Recipe #6), Whole Grain Snacks (#5), Fresh Leaf Salad (#1, with two tablespoons of peanut butter included), and an apple, is 40% more of food, it contains fewer calories, much more nutrients and fiber, while the animal-based dinner has more than triple the protein necessary for a meal and more than 11 times as much saturated fat. The low caloric density of plant-based protein makes it easier to eat a filling amount of food so you don't feel starved. Because it generally contains fewer calories per unit of weight or volume, if you want to lose weight, switching to plant protein and dropping animal protein might be the single most important food decision you can make. As we have seen, replacing most or all of the animal-based protein sources in your diet with plant-based foods like beans, fruits, nuts, vegetables, and whole grains still gives you plenty of protein to meet the minimum US RDA, safeguards your health, and has enormous potential to make your body leaner, stronger, and healthier over the long term by giving you better nutrition for fewer calories.

Especially relevant – considering the pervasiveness of obesity – is evidence showing that people eating vegan foods lose weight more effectively, even compared to those who follow a traditional low-saturated-fat "heart smart" diet. A study published in late 2005 followed 64 overweight middle-aged women assigned to either a traditional low-cholesterol diet or a low-fat vegan diet. Neither group was told to count calories or limit portion sizes. While the first group's low-cholesterol diet was what you might very reasonably think of as healthy, with "heart smart" foods like lean meat, low-fat dairy, and fish, in addition to fruits and vegetables, the second group who followed a vegan diet of beans, fruits, nuts, vegetables, and whole grains and eliminated all animal-based food completely did better. Both groups lost weight over the 14 weeks of the study, but the vegan group did lost an average of 13 pounds, 63 percent more than the average 8 pounds lost by the traditional "healthy foods" group.[332] The study's authors suggested that the difference in part might be because vegan foods digest more slowly by the body and at greater caloric cost. The protein in plant-based food comes in a healthier package.

Step 7: Use Supplements Skeptically

Focusing on the fundamentals – getting vigorous exercise in a variety of forms, eating a varied diet of healthy food, and making time for sufficient and restful sleep – is probably more important than what supplements you take. Excluding from consideration powerful hormonal supplements like steroids and their long-term health effects (and the legal and ethical muddiness of using substances that are often banned), four supplements stand out as having some evidentiary support, especially for vegans: a standard-dose multivitamin multi-mineral supplement, vegan glucosamine, HMB, and creatine.

While outright vitamin or mineral deficiency remains rare, at least in developed countries, you might nevertheless now and then be getting less than you need. As insurance against this kind of marginal deficiency, take a multivitamin every day.[345] This advice is particularly relevant for vegans, for whom vitamin B12, which comes only from bacteria that live in the soil or the digestive tracts of animals, is the only nutrient consistently missing from a strictly plant-sourced diet.[346, 347] Recent work has found that vegans who eschew multivitamins and do not include food like B12-fortified nutritional yeast in their diet do develop a measurable deficiency.[348, 349, 350] Taking a daily multivitamin will ensure you get enough. What kind of multivitamin is best? A typical multivitamin should work fine as long as it follows the standards formulated by the United States Pharmacopeia, or "USP." In addition to vitamin B12, each USP-labeled multivitamin contains vitamins A, B6, C, D, E, and K, as well as the vitamins biotin, folate, niacin, pantothenic acid, riboflavin, and thiamine, and the minerals boron, calcium, chloride, chromium, iodide, iron, magnesium, manganese, molybdenum, nickel, phosphorus, potassium, selenium, silicon, tin, and vanadium in the tiny amounts established by the USP to be more than adequate for over 90 percent of the population. More is not necessarily better. Vitamins and minerals compete for absorption, so larger doses of any one specific nutrient can interfere with the absorption of others. At dosages beyond the recommended amount, a vitamin or mineral has no greater effectiveness and can even become counterproductive, as is the case with antioxidants which at even moderately high doses start to act as free radicals[351] implicated in the aging process.[352] Follow the advice of the USP and the Harvard School of Public Health,[353] not supplement manufacturers, and take a normal, not a mega, daily multivitamin.

An unavoidable fact of life is the slow deterioration of joint cartilage over the years: by age 65, some 80 percent of us will show evidence of arthritis on x-ray.[354] An unequivocally effective supplement to enhance or protect joint cartilage has yet to be found, but there is some evidence that glucosamine, an amino sugar used to maintain and protect joint cartilage, may temper arthritis pain and possibly slow joint deterioration. A trial of 212 patients taking 1.5 grams of glucosamine daily over three years showed 80 percent less joint space narrowing on x-ray compared to placebo.[355] Another trial of 200 patients with knee arthritis also taking 1.5 grams glucosamine daily for three years also showed that while the placebo group lost 0.19 millimeters of joint space, the glucosamine group gained 0.4 millimeters.[356] A third trial of 1,583 patients with knee arthritis combining 1.5 grams of glucosamine with 1.2 grams chondroitin showed reduced arthritis pain compared to placebo, although not reduced enough to be statistically significant (in other words, the amount of pain reduction was less than that which could be attributable to chance), except for people with moderate-to-severe knee arthritis pain, for whom the glucosamine-chondroitin supplementation did show pain reduction that was both effective and statistically significant.[357] Based on these promising findings, the large-scale National Institutes of Health Glucosamine-Chondroitin Arthritis Intervention Trial (GAIT) study was launched in 2002. It showed that significant reduction in joint pain did occur for those with moderate-to-severe knee arthritis, but no other positive results.[358,359] Post-GAIT study research analyzed six more studies, two of them on glucosamine and four on chondroitin, a total of 1,502 cases, and found the evidence showed glucosamine-chondroitin supplementation over two or three years can, if only slightly, slow the knee arthritis progression on x-ray.[360] Evidence like this suggests that daily supplementation with 1.5 grams glucosamine and 1 gram chondroitin appears to be safe and at least somewhat effective for lessening arthritis pain and joint damage.

A problem with chondroitin is that it can only be manufactured from animal sources, like pig, cow, or, even less acceptably, shark cartilage. Only glucosamine is currently available in vegan form. You don't have to be vegan, I think, to find the meager added benefit afforded by chondroitin poor justification for the destruction of animals, particularly endangered ones like sharks. Those concerned with reducing animal suffering and avoiding the introduction of animal-based products into their bodies might take heart (and save money) from the multiple, if conflicting,[361] findings demonstrating reduction of arthritis-related joint destruction from glucosamine alone, at least until a cost-effective way is found to derive chondroitin from plant-based sources. Summing up much of the evidence on glucosamine and chondroitin (as well as other anti-arthritis interventions like avocado-soybean unsaponifiables, diacerein, and hyaluronic acid injection) is a well-researched critical review from Creighton University: it concludes that even though the data remains conflicting, the benefits questionable, and the promise elusive, the best evidence is for glucosamine.[362] So, some prevention of arthritis is better than none.

A stronger case exists for creatine, a nitrogen-containing organic compound synthesized by your body from amino acids. Your muscles use it to store phosphate, and rapidly burn creatine along with other phosphate-related compounds for quick energy during high-demand activity such as strength training or plyometrics. For quick access, your body concentrates creatine and other phosphate compounds in fast-twitch muscle fibers.[363] Researchers think creatine might increase the size of muscles by helping them retain water. While not every study has shown a statistically measurable benefit, a review of some 22 published studies concluded that strength training combined with creatine supplementation results in a performance gain averaging 14 percent over strength training alone.[364] Furthermore, even though the body synthesizes about one gram of creatine daily, primarily in the kidneys, liver, and pancreas,[365] creatine does not exist in plant-based foods, so the case for creatine supplementation might be stronger for vegans.[366]

How much creatine should you take? Most of the studies show positive effects on strength and lean muscle mass with a daily dose of five grams – about one and a half teaspoons – although half of that amount has been found to be equally effective.[367] Since no evidence suggests that taking a greater amount of creatine has a greater effect, you could simply take five grams daily for the first week to load creatine into your system, and then drop to half that dose in subsequent weeks. Sugar enhances creatine absorption, but as there's little evidence that creatine absorption is a problem for most people, and the sugar would also give you unnecessary calories, ingest plain creatine at mealtime to take advantage of the sugars already present in your food.

Performance improvements related to creatine have only been reported for intense exercise,[368] so creatine supplementation probably would not make much difference for exercisers doing primarily walking and limited strength activity. Similarly, there appears to be little benefit from taking creatine when you are training for endurance rather than for intensity or power.[369] Also keep in mind that by periodically going without the supplement, you might help promote your body's ability to manufacture creatine on its own. Blood plasma measurements of athletes who used creatine supplements showed that they still carried creatine in their bloodstreams even 30 days after they stopped taking the supplement.[370] So consider taking a month off from creatine supplementation now and then, particularly in periods when you're focused on endurance instead of strength. Finally, if you use creatine, abstain from caffeine (which itself seems to help facilitate burning fat during exercise[371] and increases endurance exercise tolerance,[372] although not in habitual users[373]), as simultaneous creatine and caffeine use results in caffeine totally negating creatine's ergogenic (work and strength building) effects.[374]

While supplements can give you a small edge, the real adventure in any lifelong nutrition effort is in making food tasty, interesting, and fulfilling. The next section will show you how.

Section 4

THE
RECIPES

D erived solely from beans, fruits, nuts, vegetables, and whole grains, each one of these 30 easy recipes delivers a stream of satisfying, high-quality energy to power you through the day on fewer calories. They usually take less than an hour to make, and use ingredients available in most supermarkets. Some dishes, like the Energizer Oat Breakfast and Fresh Leaf Salad, are "live," which means they undergo no cooking, which many people believe degrades nutrient potency. Others, like Shepherd's Pie or Garden Vegetable Pizza, reinterpret traditional comfort food in new and healthier ways. It takes three months to go through these recipes, which, not coincidentally, is the same length as the three-month workout cycle. Try making the main recipes one cycle and the alternates the next. You'll enjoy the festive dishes near the end of each cycle during spring break, longest days of summer, peak autumn, and end of the year if you sync up the cycle of recipes with the cycle of workouts and start the recipes anew the first weekend of every January, April, July, and October. Think of these recipes as a springboard to more healthful eating for you and your family.

A few tips for putting together healthy meals for the week.

- *Buy organic.* Even though I didn't write the word "organic" in front of every recipe ingredient because it would have taken up too much space, buy and use organic ingredients whenever you can. Organic food does cost more, but it's grown without pesticides or other synthetic additives, and it contains less pesticide residue.[375,376] If it's too much to buy everything organic, at least try to buy organically farmed versions of the "dirty dozen" foods found to have the highest pesticide levels when conventionally grown, which are: apples, bell peppers, blueberries, celery, cucumbers, grapes, greens of any kind including kale and spinach, green beans, nectarines, peaches, strawberries, and potatoes.[377] Even if an ingredient you're looking for isn't on the "dirty dozen" list, you might want to buy it organic anyway because the safe level of pesticide intake isn't really known. When you buy organic, you are not only helping your own health, but the health of others: as more of us choose organically grown food, more growers will shift to organic farming. Organic farms are more likely to maintain natural areas like fence rows, to grow forage crops, and to protect environmentally sensitive areas like wetlands. Spending on organically produced food is somewhat like voting, week after week, for a cleaner earth as well as a healthier you. Your organic food dollar incentivizes growers to devise organic production methods for farming other crops, like the cotton that most experts thought until just recently could only be grown conventionally. Some of this research has resulted in unexpected benefits, like an ongoing 30-year experiment that is suggesting that organic farming can produce hardier crops that hold up better during drought.[378] For all these reasons, going organic, like going vegan, is helpful for the world as well as for your body.

- *Ease in to eating this way.* The diet created by these recipes might best be adopted gradually, not all at once. Plant tissue relies on indigestible cellulose for much of its structure. This indigestibility is inherent to some of the salutary properties of the plant diet like its slower rate of conversion to energy, and its ability to satiate at a lower caloric intake. If you're used to the low fiber and easy digestibility of a diet high in animal and processed food, you might want to change gradually to give yourself time to get used to the gastrointestinal volatility[379] you might experience as you adjust to a plant-based way of eating. There doesn't seem to be any research on the optimal rate of change from partial to totally plant-derived cuisine, but common sense might suggest using the same rate of change we used for converting an all-walking cardio workout to an all-jogging one, or 10 percent per week. This would mean starting out just replacing 10 percent of your food with whole-food vegan recipes, and adding another 10 percent chunk each week so that by 10 weeks you're eating totally vegan.

- *Getting the amounts right.* The cookware list below and the recipes that follow are sized for two average adults with good appetites, but it also works pretty well for a single-person household as well. As you get used to preparing the food, you can adjust the portions to fit your needs. Couples might end up finishing some of the bean-based dishes or salad before the week is over, if that's the case, no problem, a good standby bean-based dish is prepared beans (Recipe #4) with canned soup, your fix of healthy greens can be met in a pinch with frozen greens seasoned with a little whole sugar, sesame seed, and soy sauce. Or use the occasion to eat out or eat at a friend's house. Singles might end up having a little extra of each, a great excuse to invite someone over and share your cooking!

- *Have essential cookware.* All you need to cook every one of the recipes in this book are: a (6-quart) pressure cooker, a food processor, a large chef's knife, a small chef's knife, a knife sharpener, a set of long wooden spoons, a long wooden ladle, a handheld garlic press, a handheld grater, a small mist sprayer bottle (like Tolco Neon mist spray bottle), a wheeled pizza cutter, a large wooden cutting board, a large (6- or 7-quart) stockpot, a medium (3-quart) soup pot, and a large (10-inch) frying pan (Caraway cookware sells a nicely non-toxic non-stick set of these items as a 6.5-quart Dutch oven, a 10.5-inch fry pan, and a 3-quart sauce pan, plus a 4.5-quart sauté pan), a small (1-quart) sauce pan, two large foil baking trays, long wooden spoons, a can opener, a drainer, a hand-held mesh sieve, a wide pancake turner, aluminum foil, two large aluminum foil trays, a pair of oven gloves or potholders, three very large (17-cup), eight large (12-cup), three medium (a 10-cup, and 8-cup, and a 6-cup, or similar), one small (3-cup), and one very small (1-cup) food storage containers, and heavy duty sponges. Good, high-quality (*non-toxic* non-stick, like Caraway) cookware might cost a little more but it will heat better and last longer. This saves you labor and money in the long run.

- *Rely on primary foods.* You don't have to make every dish a masterpiece. The recipes in this book build a simple but healthy cuisine from five easy-to-make foods, each designated as a "primary food," that together complement each other while giving you a solid nutritional base. The recipes will show you how to start each day out with a breakfast of leaf salad (Recipe #1, Fresh Leaf Salad), a root salad (Recipe #2, Root Pieces), and a delicious, no-cooking-required cereal (Recipe #3, Energizer Breakfast). For lunch, have beans (Recipe #4, Beans Four Ways), a grain dish, and more fresh salad (Recipe #1 again), and for dinner, a bean dish along with a tasty snack of whole-grained chips (Recipe #7, Whole Grain Snacks), and still another bowl of fresh salad, this time topped with a fillip of nut butter (Recipe #1, Fresh Leaf Salad, a third time). By being easy to make, these primary foods make sustainable a dietary approach that displaces less healthy foods off of your menu.

- *Branch out, pairing beans with grains.* Each week, choose a bean dish from the even-numbered recipes on the even-numbered (left-side) pages, and make it over the weekend, and have it as your bean dish for supper. Also each week, pick a grain dish from the odd-numbered recipes on the odd-numbered (right-side) pages. You usually can make the bean dish over the weekend, and also over the weekend complete the usually minimal grain dish preparation. Then during the week, you can rather quickly cook up a serving-sized portion of the grain dish each morning to have ready for lunch, and treat yourself to a helping of the bean dish for supper. The recipes will show you how.

- *Shop once a week.* If you've retired in a French village where the grocery store is a picturesque community meeting space, go ahead and shop for fresh ingredients daily, but most of us can save time by doing the food shopping once a week.

- *Use a list.* Food shopping is easy with a grocery list. Try keeping at least two of any staple (non-perishable) item, so whenever you run out of one, write it on the list. That way, you have all week to use the other one without running out.

- *Prepare over the weekend.* Each week, pick two recipes (one bean, one grain) you think you'd like to try for the coming week, and write their ingredients on the list, plus the ingredients for the salads (Recipe #1, Fresh Leaf Salad, and Recipe #2, Root Pieces). Many of the recipes can be prepared, often completely, ahead of time over the weekend so that you can enjoy fresh home-made food without having to do a lot of food preparation during the week. Cooking takes time but can also be a great way to unwind.

- *Adjust your portions to you.* Use the girth measurement method (page 11) to assess how well this way of eating is working for you. One of the benefits of eating vegan is that if you're trying to lose weight, you may not have to strive as hard to control portions as you would with less healthy food. A serving of a dish should usually be no bigger than the size of your closed fist. Portions also should be, well, in proportion. For example, the grain-based portions should be roughly the size of the bean-based and salad-based portions, not multiple times larger.

- *Share.* Food shopping, cooking, and meals can be "you" time but also are times for family and friends. As you get more familiar with cooking, pass the results of your efforts around a lively table.

Okay, let's get started making some good food.

1. Fresh Leaf Salad primary food

The cornerstone of healthful eating, this versatile salad has ingredients that should survive an entire week of refrigeration without losing their freshness. Enjoy the subtle, complex, and even bitter flavors of the diverse ingredients, knowing that they help your health. You can eat this salad with your hands, just like you would do with chips. Have some of this salad with every meal – including breakfast – to increase your nutrient and fiber intake without driving up calorie consumption.

12 robust refrigeration-resilient salad greens like baby broccoli (broccolini), broccoli rabe, celery, collard greens, dandelion greens (red and white), kale (green, lanceolate, and red), purple cabbage, Swiss chard (rainbow, red, and white), and turnip greens
1 or 2 packages of fresh herbs like dill, mint, parsley, sage, or tarragon

Each weekend, slice or chop each ingredient and distribute among 6 large (12-cup) food containers and refrigerate. Every meal, have a large serving, including breakfast.

NUT BUTTER VARIATION   At dinner, have a spoonful or two — maximum — of 100% nut butter (like Teddy's Super Chunky All Natural Peanut Butter) along with the salad.

2. Beet Shreds primary food

Breakfast curbs your appetite, raises your metabolism, is more likely to be burned off than food eaten later, and people who eat breakfast lose weight more easily.[380] Start your day with this beautifully simple shredded salad made from colorful beets, carrots, and radishes.

1 or 2 golden beets
1 or 2 red-and-white (Chioggia) beets (optional)
1 or 2 regular (purple) beets
4 to 6 carrots
1 bunch radishes
lemon juice

Over the weekend, wash and remove any leaves or root tips from golden beets, red-and-white Chioggia beets (optional), regular (purple) beets, carrots, radishes, and refrigerate. Fill a small spray bottle (like Tolco's neon mist sprayer) with lemon juice and refrigerate. Each morning make a small fresh salad by grating a little of each root vegetable into a small dish using a handheld grater, and spritz with lemon juice.

TURNIP VARIATION   Grate fennel, jicama, parsnips, rutabaga, turnip and spray with lime juice.

3. Energizer Oat Breakfast primary food

Cold water is, surprisingly, all you need to unlock the whole grain sweetness of this dish that complements the preceding leaf and root salads to make a complete breakfast. It's vital to get raisins that are juicy, the only source of which as of this writing (August, 2023), seems to be Sun-Maid raisins in 12-ounce bags sold on Amazon. With the sweetness of the raisins, you'll be fine with just chilled water!

¼ cup old-fashioned oats
¼ cup whole grain cereal (like Post's Grape-Nuts)
¼ cup a second whole grain cereal (like Nature's Path Heritage Flakes)
1 tablespoon mixed nuts
¼ cup jumbo mixed raisins (like Sun-Maid Mixed Jumbo Raisins, Large Raisin Medley Includes Golden Raisins and Red Flame Raisins)

Each morning, place old-fashioned oats, whole grain cereals (like Post's Grape-Nuts), mixed nuts, and jumbo mixed raisins (like Sun-Maid Mixed Jumbo Raisins, Large Raisin Medley Includes Golden Raisins and Red Flame Raisins) in a bowl and serve. Add chilled water as needed. Have each morning for breakfast. The first weekend before you make this cereal, buy two containers of each dry ingredient. Whenever you finish a container, write it on your grocery list. That way, you can wait until the next weekend's food shopping to replenish it without running out. Prepare this breakfast only shortly before serving. Or mix the dry ingredients together to take to work or wherever, and add the water only shortly before serving.

FURTHER VARIATION Try adding different whole grain cereals (but read the nutrition facts on the boxes first and avoid ones high in added sugars or sweeteners), sparing amounts of different juices (stick with ones 100% derived from fruit without added sugars or sweeteners), or plant-based milks (again avoiding ones with added sugars or sweeteners).

4. Beans Four Ways primary food

Using a pressure cooker makes bean preparation easy. You don't even need to soak the beans, just rinse them. A fascinating investigation, by the enterprising J. Kenji López-Alt of the Serious Eats blog, involved experimentally feeding beans prepared various ways to the family dog. It concluded that soaking beans provides no benefit and only drains away color, flavor, and nutritive properties.[381] In a hurry? Use canned beans instead, which need no rinsing. Make this nutritionally sound bean dish part of your daily lunch, spiced up with a home-made seasoning salt, which, with its ratio of one-part salt to seven parts other spices — 87% less sodium — can be substituted for the coarse salt used in many of the recipes that follow. Avoiding smaller beans like lentils or split peas, which have an unfortunate tendency to dissolve into goo, I like a mix of eight beans commonly available in single packages: black beans, black-eyed peas, chick peas, great northern beans, kidney beans, large lima beans, navy beans, and pinto beans. Nearly every bean recipe in this book uses 2½ cups of dry beans, equivalent to one 16-ounce package.

2½ cups (or 16 oz) of mixed beans like black beans, black-eyed peas, chick peas, great northern beans, kidney beans, large lima beans, navy beans, pinto beans, or try heirloom beans like appaloosa, borlatti, Christmas lima, cranberry, flageolet, marcella, scarlet runner, vaquero, or yellow eye beans

½ teaspoon home-made seasoning salt (equal parts coarse salt, celery seed, smoked paprika, coarse black pepper, dried mustard powder, dried onion granules, dried parsley, and turmeric)

Over the weekend, rinse a wide variety of mixed beans in the drainer, place in the pressure cooker, adding three times as much water as beans, close and seal, and set to cook for 1 hour and 30 minutes. Let cool and refrigerate in a storage container. Prepare a home-made seasoning salt of equal parts coarse salt, celery seed, smoked paprika (only smoked paprika has a beautifully bright red color), coarse black pepper, dried mustard powder, dried onion granules, dried parsley, and turmeric. In the morning for lunch, scoop out a serving of beans and sprinkle on a little of the home-made seasoning salt.

FOUR SIMPLE VARIATIONS Place the rinsed beans in the pressure cooker, adding three times as much water as beans, close and seal, and set to cook for 1 hour and 20 minutes. Spice up the beans with a little coarse salt and pepper. Or salt and French *herbes de Provence* (marjoram, oregano, rosemary, summer savory, and thyme) seasoning. Or salt and Lebanese seven spices (allspice, black pepper, cinnamon, ground cloves, coriander, cumin, and nutmeg) seasoning. Or try the zen-like simplicity of having the beans plain with no seasoning at all.

5. **Whole Grain Snacks** primary food

If you stick to the rest of the diet in this book, you should be able to guiltlessly enjoy this easy-to-make whole grain vegan snack medley with your evening meal. Just look for the yellow and brown Whole Grain logo (except for pretzels, I have yet to find a decent whole-grain pretzel) and make sure there's no added cheese, other dairy, hydrogenated oil, or sugar. On movie night, make home-made popcorn instead.

a few each of whole grain vegan snacks like Garden of Eatin's Multi-Grain Chips, Kraft's Original Corn Nuts, Late July's How Sweet Potato It Is Tortilla Chips, Lundberg's Sea Salt Rice Chips, Mary's Gone Crackers Original Crackers, Nabisco's Garden Herb Triscuits, or Zack's Mighty Tortilla Chips

Over the weekend, get whole grain vegan snacks like Garden of Eatin's Multi-Grain Chips, Kraft's Original Corn Nuts, Late July's How Sweet Potato It Is Tortilla Chips, Lundberg's Sea Salt Rice Chips, Mary's Gone Crackers Original Crackers, Nabisco's Garden Herb Triscuits, or Zack's Mighty Tortilla Chip. Each night before dinner, just put a few (3 to 5) chips or crackers from each into a small bowl and serve. Keep the bags closed so the chips don't get stale or pick up humidity from the surrounding air.

HOME-MADE POPCORN VARIATION   Once in a while, make popcorn by placing popcorn kernels in a medium-sized soup pot along with oil (throughout these recipes, use canola oil interchangeably with other low-saturated-fat, mild-flavored, sustainably sourced plant-based cooking oils like grapeseed, safflower, or sunflower oil — never palm oil), cover, apply high heat until the kernels stop popping, empty into a large bowl, garnish with coarse salt and extra virgin olive oil.

6. Minestrone

We begin a three-month cycle of pairing bean-based dishes (here on the even-numbered, left-side pages) with grain dishes (on the odd-numbered, right-side pages). Each weekend, make a bean dish and a grain dish for the week: have the bean dish (with Whole Grain Snacks) for supper, and the grain dish (with Beans Four Ways) for lunch, along with Fresh Leaf Salad, which you should have with every meal. Instead of large portions, sate your appetite with an apple as a nighttime dessert. This recipe, a venerable vegan tradition predating Roman times, is, like all the bean stew recipes in this book, made easy using a pressure cooker.

2½ cups (or one 16-ounce package) of any kind of dry beans
1 (16-ounce) can cooked beans (any kind)
3 carrots
1 (8-ounce) package fresh green beans
1 onion
1 head garlic
1 (15-ounce) can cooked beans, any kind
1 (28-ounce) can crushed tomatoes
1 bunch fresh parsley
½ tablespoon French *herbes de Provence* seasoning

Rinse a package of dry beans (any kind) and place in a pressure cooker, along with a can of cooked beans (any kind), diced carrots, chopped fresh green beans (ends removed), peeled diced onion, peeled and pressed garlic, canned crushed tomatoes, finely sliced fresh parsley, dried French *herbes de Provence* seasoning, and water almost to the fill line. Seal and cook for 1 hour and 30 minutes.

BORSCHT VARIATION   Rinse a package of the dry beans (any kind) and place in pressure cooker, along with a can of cooked beans (any kind), diced beet (any kind), carrots, zucchini, onion, canned crushed tomatoes, canned diced tomatoes, dried dill, and water almost to the fill line. Seal and cook for 1 hour and 30 minutes.

7. Cornmeal-Crusted Soy Steak Sandwich

These nice sourdough sandwiches kick off a series of grain-based lunch dishes that go well with the preceding Beans Four Ways and Fresh Leaf Salad to make a complete lunch.

aioli
¼ **cup vegan mayonnaise (like Plant Perfect's Vegan Mayo with no Palm Oil Ever)**
2 garlic cloves
2 teaspoons sesame oil
1 tablespoon grated lemon rind
¼ **cup fresh parsley**

1 teaspoon cornmeal
1 teaspoon dried minced onion
½ **teaspoon dried basil**
3 slices of (14-ounce) package extra-firm tofu
3 slices of sliced sourdough artisan bread
2 teaspoons oil
3 leaves of dark greens like collard, dandelion, or kale
3 slices of fresh tomato

Over the weekend, freeze a loaf of sourdough artisan bread being sure not to squeeze the slices together. Each morning, lightly toast 3 slices of the bread (or bake 5 minutes at 350° on a foil tray), mix a little cornmeal, dried minced onion, and dried basil in a bowl, and in another bowl an aioli of vegan mayonnaise (like Plant Perfect's Vegan Mayo with no Palm Oil Ever), freshly pressed garlic, sesame oil, freshly grated lemon rind, and fresh parsley, slice off 3 thin pieces of the tofu, add oil to a frying pan, sprinkle one-half of the cornmeal mixture over the oil, add the 3 tofu slices, fry on medium heat a few minutes, flip, sprinkle with rest of the cornmeal mixture, add 3 leaves of dark greens, fry another minute, turn off heat. Layer bread, aioli, soy steak, a thin slice of fresh tomato, dark greens, the second piece of bread, slice sandwich in half and serve.

WATERCRESS GINGER WALNUT VARIATION Over the weekend, freeze the loaf of sliced sourdough artisan bread being sure not to squeeze the slices together. When ready to make the sandwiches, toast 3 slices of the bread (or bake at 350° 5 minutes on a foil tray). Add some oil, onion and walnuts to a frying pan on medium heat a few minutes until onions softened, add some freshly grated ginger root and balsamic vinegar, turn off heat. Layer the toasted bread with the cooked onion filling, some fresh watercress, the second piece of bread, slice sandwich in half and serve.

8. Cassoulet

This stew cheerfully discards the meat while reverently preserving the classic herbal flavors of this traditional French casserole.

2½ dry white beans (any kind, like navy, white kidney, great northern, or cannellini)
1 (15-ounce) can baked beans (like Whole Foods' Maple and Onion Baked Beans)
3 stalks celery
1 onion
1 head garlic
1 (15-ounce) can cooked squash
1 (14-ounce) can diced tomatoes
1 bunch fresh sage
1 tablespoon lemon juice
2 teaspoons dried tarragon
2 teaspoons dried thyme
1 teaspoon coarse black pepper

Over the weekend, rinse a package of dry white beans (any kind of white beans, like navy, white kidney, great northern, or cannellini) and place in pressure cooker along with a can of cooked baked beans (like Whole Foods' Maple & Onion Baked Beans), celery, onion, peeled and pressed garlic, canned cooked squash, canned diced tomatoes, fresh sage, lemon juice, dried tarragon, dried thyme, coarse black pepper, and water almost to the fill line. Seal and cook for 1 hour and 30 minutes.

ORANGE MARMALADE VARIATION Over the weekend, rinse a package of dry white beans (any kind) and place in pressure cooker along with a can of cooked baked beans (like Whole Foods' Maple & Onion Baked Beans), cucumber, orange or red bell pepper, canned diced tomatoes, canned cooked pumpkin, fresh tarragon, apple cider vinegar, summer savory, dried thyme, and water almost to the fill line. Seal and cook for 1 hour and 30 minutes. Before serving, top with a spritz of an orange marmalade.

9. Whole Grain Biscuits

Grain as it was meant to be, with bran and germ intact. Higher whole grain consumption continues to relate to lower risk of cardiovascular disease, diabetes, and multiple types of cancer.[382] Pair large-size whole grains like hulled barley, brown rice, buckwheat groats, farro, kamut, spelt berries, rye, wheat (hard red, hard red spring, hard white, or soft white), or triticale with whole grain flours from amaranth, brown rice, buckwheat, corn (blue, white, or yellow), graham, millet, quinoa, rye, sorghum, spelt, teff, triticale, or whole wheat. I like to pair whole wheat flour with a 7-grain mix of whole brown rice, buckwheat, chickpea, corn, millet, oat, rye, and spelt flours.

¼ cup large-size whole grain like barley, brown rice, buckwheat groats, farro, kamut, spelt, rye, wheat, or triticale (two kinds are nice)
½ cup whole wheat flour
½ cup whole grain flour
½ teaspoon baking powder
½ teaspoon coarse salt

In a small saucepan toast large-size whole grains on medium heat 5 minutes until grain aromatic. Spray oil on a sheet of foil. I like to place a large foil tray under the foil sheet, that way crumbs and oil don't end up on the bottom of the oven. Mix whole wheat flour, whole grain flour, the toasted grain, (aluminum-free) baking powder, coarse salt, add only enough water to make a shapeable dough, form into two or three small biscuits, transfer to the oil-sprayed foil on foil tray, bake 350° 20 minutes until crust golden-brown. Serve with a little no-palm-oil vegan butter, like Miyoko's Butter.

WHOLE GRAIN BREAD VARIATION The secret to good yeast proofing is getting the water just hot enough. Since it's a lot easier to cool water down than to warm it up, use this method to adjust the water temperature: warm ⅓ cup water in microwave 30 seconds, adding a little cold water if needed until water is uncomfortably yet tolerably hot to your fingers - if your fingers can't tolerate the heat, neither will your yeast. Add a pinch of whole sugar (like Wholesome's Sucanat), a spoonful of yeast, stir, and set aside to proof. Toast whole grain in a small saucepan on high heat until aromatic. Place foil sheet on a foil tray, spray sheet with oil, place spoonful whole grain flour on cutting board, place a spoonful extra virgin olive oil in small bowl. Mix whole wheat flour, whole grain flour, the toasted grains, coarse salt, and enough yeast and water mixture to make a shapeable dough, shape into a ball, coat with the whole grain flour, then the extra virgin olive oil, and transfer to the oil-sprayed foil on foil tray, put bread and foil on a foil tray, pour oil from bowl atop, bake 350° 25 minutes until crust golden-brown. Serve with a little no-palm-oil vegan butter (like Miyoko's Butter).

10. **Provincial Veggie Stew**

Two simple bean-based stews make a comforting, nourishing dinnertime meal with flavors of the countryside.

2½ cups (one 16-ounce package) dry beans, any kind
1 (15-ounce) can cooked beans, any kind
2 carrots
2 stalks celery
1 onion
1 (6-ounce) can tomato paste
1 (16-ounce) package frozen green peas
2 teaspoons garlic powder
1 teaspoon coarse black pepper
1 (16-ounce) container vegetable broth (like Whole Food's Veggie Broth)

Into a pressure cooker, place dry beans (any kind), canned cooked beans (any kind), carrots, celery, onion, tomato paste, frozen green peas, whole grain flour, garlic powder, black pepper, and vegetable broth (like Whole Food's Veggie Broth), add water almost to the fill line, seal, and cook for 1 hour and 30 minutes.

HERBES DE PROVENCE VARIATION   Into a pressure cooker, place dry beans (any kind), canned cooked beans (any kind), carrots, celery, onion, peeled and pressed garlic, tomatoes, fresh parsley, French *herbes de Provence* (marjoram, oregano, rosemary, summer savory, and thyme) seasoning, and vegetable broth (like Whole Food's Veggie Broth), add water almost to the fill line, seal, and cook for 1 hour and 30 minutes.

11. Burgers and "Fries"

Two delicious burgers, one from black beans, the other from the versatile red lentil, go along with home-made not-fried "fries" in these vegan takes on the All-American lunch.

4 cups (five 15-ounce cans) cooked black beans
½ teaspoon oil
1 green bell pepper
1 onion
8 garlic cloves
½ cup ground flaxseed
1 (12-ounce) package vegan mozzarella cheese (like Violife's Vegan Mozzarella)
1 bunch fresh parsley
1 tablespoon ketchup
½ teaspoon chili powder
½ teaspoon cumin
½ teaspoon dried garlic granules
½ teaspoon smoked paprika
2 packages whole grain hamburger buns
Romaine lettuce, fresh tomatoes, and mustard

potatoes, oil, and coarse salt

Over the weekend, freeze the whole grain buns. Drain and rinse five cans of cooked black beans. In a large stockpot over medium heat place oil, the black beans, green bell pepper, onion, peeled and pressed garlic, stir, and turn off heat. Add ground flaxseed, vegan mozzarella cheese (like Violife's Vegan Mozzarella), fresh parsley, ketchup, chili powder, cumin, dried garlic granules, smoked paprika, and stir. Refrigerate. Before serving, make the "fries" by cutting up one or two potatoes, place in a plastic bag along with some oil and coarse salt, shake, pour out onto an oil-sprayed foil tray, and roast at 350° 45 minutes until crispy but not burnt. Place each patty in large frying pan with oil on medium heat, sizzle and flip. Place each bun in oven on a foil tray, toast at 350° five minutes. Layer bottom bun, burger, sliced onion, tomato, lettuce, mustard, and top bun.

RED LENTIL VARIATION Over weekend, place 1:1 red lentils to water in pressure cooker, seal and cook for 5 minutes, unseal and chopped onion, pressed garlic, grated carrot, fresh parsley, tomato paste, coarse black pepper, blend, and refrigerate. Before serving, cut up one or two potatoes, place in a plastic bag along with some oil and coarse salt, shake, put on an oil-sprayed foil tray, and roast at 350° 45 minutes until crispy but not burnt. Place each patty in large frying pan with oil on medium heat, sizzle and flip. Place each bun in oven on a foil tray, toast at 350° five minutes. Layer bottom bun, burger, sliced onion, tomato, Romaine lettuce, ketchup, and top bun.

12. Golden Split Pea Stew

Simmering peacefully in the pressure cooker, the yellow split peas in both the apple and peach versions of this stew merge into a golden ambrosia.

2½ cups (one 16-ounce package) yellow split peas
2 apples
2 carrots
1 onion
3 cloves garlic
2 fresh ginger roots
1 bunch Swiss chard
2 teaspoons fresh lemon juice
1 (14-ounce) can diced tomatoes
1 teaspoon dried thyme
½ teaspoon turmeric

Into a pressure cooker, place dry yellow split peas, apples, onion, peeled and pressed garlic, finely diced fresh ginger, finely chopped Swiss chard, lemon juice, canned diced tomatoes, dried thyme, dried turmeric, and water almost to the fill line, seal and cook for 1 hour and 15 minutes.

PEACH VARIATION Into a pressure cooker, place dry yellow split peas, frozen peaches, carrots, scallions (save one or two from the bunch to use in the next recipe, Shepherd's Pie), finely diced fresh ginger, canned cooked pumpkin, finely chopped Swiss chard, lemon juice, canned diced tomatoes, and water almost to the fill line, seal and cook for 1 hour and 15 minutes.

13. Shepherd's Pie

Simple biscuits surround this comforting shepherd's pie and the festive corn tamale variation.

filling
1 potato
2 carrots
½ (12-ounce) package frozen green peas
1 teaspoon celery seed
1 teaspoon smoked paprika

biscuit
½ cup whole wheat flour
½ cup whole grain flour
1 teaspoon coarse salt
2 teaspoons oil

Over the weekend, microwave potato and carrots 2 minutes at a time several times until soft, let cool, and refrigerate. Before serving, place foil sheet on foil tray, spray sheet with oil. Mix a filling of a little of the potato, a little of the carrot, some frozen green peas (by the end of the week have half the frozen green peas still left in the package to use in next week's Hearty Root Stew), celery seed, and smoked paprika. Mix whole wheat flour, grain flour, coarse salt, oil, and enough water to make a shapeable dough. Shape three-quarters of the dough into a little bowl, place it on the oil-sprayed foil on a foil tray, fill the bowl with the filling, shape a lid out of the remaining dough and put it on top. Bake at 350° 30 minutes until crust is golden.

CORN TAMALE VARIATION Place foil sheet on foil tray, spray sheet with oil. Mix a filling of some cashews, onion, tomatoes, a little lime juice, and chili powder. Make a dough of whole wheat flour, whole grain flour, cornmeal, coarse salt, oil, and just enough water to shape three-quarters of the dough into a little bowl, place it on the oil-sprayed foil on a foil tray, fill the bowl with the filling, shape a lid out of the remaining dough and put it on top. Bake at 350° 30 minutes until crust golden.

14. Hearty Root Stew

Pasta sauce adds sweetness and depth to two more simple bean stews.

2½ cups (one 16-ounce package) any kind of dry beans
1 (15-ounce) can refried beans
1 rutabaga or turnip
3 stalks celery
1 onion
1 (14-ounce) can diced tomatoes
1 cup (½ of a 10-ounce package) frozen green peas
1 (24-ounce) jar pasta sauce (like Whole Foods' Organic Tomato and Basil Pasta Sauce)

Rinse a package of dry beans (any kind) and place in a pressure cooker along with a can of refried beans, a rutabaga or turnip, celery, onion, diced tomatoes, half a package of frozen green peas (use the rest of the green peas from last week's Shepherd's Pie recipe), pasta sauce (like Whole Foods' Organic Tomato and Basil Pasta Sauce), and water almost to the fill line. Seal and cook for 1 hour and 30 minutes.

DEEPER SHADE OF SOUL VARIATION Rinse a package of dry black-eyed peas and place in a pressure cooker along with a can of refried beans (any kind), a beet, carrot, onion, diced tomatoes, fresh thinly sliced collard greens, pasta sauce, and water almost to the fill line. Seal and cook for 1 hour and 30 minutes.

15. Flatbread Pieces

This tasty flatbread is dressed with either a tomato-basil or mushroom-red-bell-pepper topping and sweetened with malted barley flour. For dusting the cutting board, I like to use "exotic" flours like amaranth, barley, quinoa, or teff, as these are different from my 7-grain "workhorse" whole grain flour mix of bean, brown rice, buckwheat, millet, oat, rye, and spelt flours.

topping
1 tablespoon sunflower kernels
2 or 3 small Yukon Gold potatoes
2 small fresh tomatoes
extra virgin olive oil
1 small live basil plant

flatbread
½ cup whole wheat flour
½ cup whole grain flour
1 tablespoon malted barley flour (like Breadtopia Organic Diastatic Malt Powder)
¼ teaspoon coarse salt
1 tablespoon whole grain flour (for handling dough)

Over the weekend, microwave several small Yukon Gold potatoes 2 minutes at a time until soft, let cool, and refrigerate. Before serving, toast sunflower kernels (sunflower seeds without shell or hull) in a small saucepan on high heat until aromatic, place foil sheet on foil tray, spray sheet with oil, dust a cutting board with whole grain flour, mix whole wheat flour, whole grain flour, malted barley flour (like Breadtopia Organic Diastatic Malt Powder), coarse salt, the toasted sunflower kernels, and enough water to make a shapeable dough. Flatten dough onto the flour-dusted cutting board. Cut with pizza cutter into 9 pieces, transfer to oil-sprayed foil on foil tray. Top each piece with a bit of mashed potato, a piece of diced tomato, and drizzle on a little extra virgin olive oil. Bake at 350° 20 minutes, top each piece with a piece of a basil leaf. To have fresh basil, buy a small live basil plant for the week, keep it by a sunlit window, water it as needed, and harvest a basil leaf or two each day.

RED BELL PEPPER TARRAGON VARIATION   Toast sunflower kernels in a small saucepan on high heat until aromatic, place foil sheet on foil tray, spray sheet with oil, dust a cutting board with whole grain flour, mix whole wheat flour, whole grain flour, malted barley flour, coarse salt, the toasted sunflower kernels, and enough water to make a shapeable dough. Flatten dough onto the flour-dusted cutting board. Cut with pizza cutter into 9 pieces, transfer to oil-sprayed foil on foil tray. Top each piece with a slice of fresh mushroom, a piece of red pepper, and drizzle on a little extra virgin olive oil. Bake at 350° 20 minutes, top each piece with a few fresh tarragon leaves.

16. Bell Pepper Chili

We salute the carotene-, lycopene-, vitamin-C-, and color-rich bell pepper with these two chilis.

2½ cups (one 16-ounce package) dry kidney beans or other kind of dry beans
1 (16-ounce) can cooked beans
1 (15-ounce) can refried black beans
2 bell peppers of different colors
1 zucchini
1 head garlic
1 can of (15-ounce) can crushed tomatoes
1 can of (6-ounce) can tomato paste
1 bunch fresh parsley
1 tablespoon agave nectar
1 teaspoon allspice powder
1 teaspoon chili powder
1 teaspoon cocoa powder
1 teaspoon smoked paprika

Place package of any kind of dry beans, a can of cooked beans (any kind), a can of refried black beans, two bell peppers of different colors, zucchini, pressed and peeled garlic, canned crushed tomatoes, canned tomato paste, fresh parsley, agave nectar, allspice powder, chili powder, cocoa powder, smoked paprika in a pressure cooker, add water almost to the fill line, seal, and cook for 1 hour and 30 minutes.

BLACK BEAN SQUASH VARIATION Place package of dry black beans, a can of cooked beans (any kind), a can of refried pinto beans, two bell peppers of different colors, onion, pressed and peeled garlic, canned pumpkin, canned squash, canned crushed tomatoes, canned tomato paste, fresh cilantro, agave nectar, allspice powder, chili powder, smoked paprika in a pressure cooker, add water almost to the fill line, seal, and cook for 1 hour and 30 minutes.

17. **Cornbread**

Thanks to (aluminum-free) baking powder, these two breads, sweetened by applesauce and agave nectar, will rise in the moodiest of ovens. Cooking times and oven temperatures may vary. Throughout this book, I've used an electric convection oven (the upper oven of a 2019 Samsung 5.9 cu. ft. Freestanding Electric Range with Flex Duo & Dual Door in Black Stainless Steel, to be exact), but every oven is a little different, so experiment to find the baking settings, cooking times, oven temperatures that you like. A 24-ounce jar of (unsweetened) applesauce should last the week.

½ **cup whole cornmeal**
¼ **cup whole wheat flour**
¼ **cup whole grain flour**
¼ **teaspoon (aluminum-free) baking powder**
dash of coarse salt
½ **cup (unsweetened) applesauce**
2 teaspoons agave nectar
1 teaspoon apple cider vinegar
just a little unsweetened soy milk
no-palm-oil vegan butter (like Miyoko's Butter)

Place foil sheet on foil tray, spray sheet with oil. Mix whole cornmeal, whole wheat flour, whole grain flour, baking powder, coarse salt, applesauce, agave nectar, apple cider vinegar, and just enough unsweetened soy milk to make a shapeable dough. Place onto the oil-sprayed foil on foil tray and bake at 350° 25 minutes. When serving, split open and insert a dab of no-palm-oil vegan butter (like Miyoko's Butter).

CARROT CAKE VARIATION WITH VEGAN CREAM CHEESE VARIATION   When ready to make the carrot cake, place foil sheet on foil tray, spray sheet with oil, grate a tablespoon of carrot, mix whole wheat flour, whole grain flour, the grated carrot, whole sugar, baking powder, ground cinnamon, ground cloves, coarse salt, then add just enough applesauce, agave nectar, and unsweetened soy milk to make a shapeable dough. Place onto the oil-sprayed foil on foil tray and bake at 350° 25 minutes. Mix a spoonful of cream cheese by placing a dab each of powdered sugar, no-palm-oil vegan cream cheese (like Kite Hill's Plain Cream Cheese), vegan butter, and a tiny amount of apple cider vinegar, and using your fingers, mix together until smooth, then refrigerate. Remove the baked carrot cake from oven. When serving, split open and insert the cream cheese.

18. Green Split Pea Stew

Guacamole and roast garlic enrich these green split pea stews.

3 heads of garlic
1 or 2 avocados
2½ cups (one 16-ounce package) dry green split peas
1 (32-ounce) package creamy tomato basil soup (like Pacific Food's Creamy Tomato Basil Soup)
1 bunch celery
1 large onion
1 (14-ounce) can diced tomatoes
1 bunch fresh arugula
2 teaspoons nutmeg

Slice the tops off of 3 heads of garlic, place them on oil-sprayed foil, close the foil up, roast at 400° 1 hour and 30 minutes, remove from oven. Peel and pit the avocados and enough water to blend them in a food processor into a guacamole paste (I like to get two avocados as "insurance," if one of them is too over- or underripe, one will do). To the pressure cooker, add dry green split peas, one package creamy tomato basil soup (like Pacific Food's Creamy Tomato Basil Soup), celery, onion, canned diced tomatoes, fresh arugula, nutmeg, and water almost up to three-quarters full. Run fingers along bottom of cooker container to loosen the green split peas, which have a way of clumping on the bottom, seal and cook for 1 hour and 30 minutes. After cooking squeeze the cooled roasted garlic bulbs to add them, along with the guacamole, to the stew.

GREEN STEMS VARIATION Slice the tops off of 3 heads of garlic, place them on oil-sprayed foil, close the foil up, roast at 400° 1 hour and 30 minutes, turn off heat but let them stay in the oven. Peel and pit the avocados and blend them with some water in a food processor into a guacamole paste. To the pressure cooker, add dry green split peas, one package squash soup (like Pacific Food's Butternut Squash Soup), finely sliced broccolini, collard green, and kale, stems, tomatoes, fresh watercress, nutmeg, and water almost up to three-quarters full. Run fingers along bottom of cooker container to loosen the green split peas, which have a way of clumping on the bottom, seal and cook for 1 hour and 30 minutes. After cooking squeeze the cooled roasted garlic bulbs to add them, along with the guacamole, to the stew.

19. Garden Vegetable Pizza
Luscious tomato, tangy tomato paste, and caramelized onion crown a scrumptious crust.

½ tablespoon active dry yeast
1 teaspoon whole sugar (like Wholesome's Sucanat)
2 tablespoons steel-cut oats or other whole grain
2 teaspoons cornmeal
1 tablespoon whole grain flour
½ cup whole wheat flour
½ cup whole grain flour
½ teaspoon coarse salt
1/6th of a (6-ounce) can tomato paste
dash basil
dash oregano
1/6th of 1 bunch baby broccoli
1/6th of 1 (12-ounce) package fresh mushrooms
1/6th of a (14-ounce) can tomatoes
3 teaspoons extra virgin olive oil
1/6th of a large onion

Warm ⅓ cup of water in microwave 30 seconds and adjust until water very hot yet tolerable to finger immersion, add pinch of whole sugar (like Wholesome's Sucanat), a tablespoon of yeast, stir, and set aside set aside in a draft-free area for 15 minutes to proof. Toast steel-cut oats or other whole grain in small saucepan on high heat. Place foil sheet on foil tray, spray sheet with oil, sprinkle with cornmeal. Place a tablespoon of whole grain flour on a cutting board. Combine whole wheat flour, whole grain flour, coarse salt, and, removing grains from heat just as small wisps of smoke appear, add to flour, stir, and add yeast and water mixture as needed to make a wet, sticky dough. Coat the dough with the whole grain flour on the cutting board, then flatten it onto the foil tray, wash hands and flour-coated surfaces. Using toppings sparingly, layer onto dough a little canned tomato paste, basil, oregano, sliced baby broccoli, sliced mushrooms, and canned diced tomatoes. Bake at 350° 20 minutes or until dough baked through. While pizza bakes, sauté onion in extra virgin olive oil on high heat just a minute or two or until edges sear, add onion and oil to top of pizza when done. Slice in four and serve.

SPINACH VARIATION   Make pizza exact same way except substitute fresh spinach for the baby broccoli and vegan mozzarella cheese shreds (like Violife's Just Like Mozzarella Shreds) for the sliced mushrooms.

20. Garden Vegetable Stew

These refreshing garden vegetable stews feature fresh cauliflower and cherry tomatoes.

2½ cups (one 16-ounce package) dry white beans, any kind
1 (15-ounce) can cooked white beans, any kind
1 head cauliflower
1 large onion
6 cloves garlic
1 (15-ounce) package cherry tomatoes
1 (6-ounce) can tomato paste
1 bunch fresh parsley
2 teaspoons cumin
1 teaspoon smoked paprika
1 teaspoon summer savory

To a pressure cooker, add dry white beans (any kind), a can of cooked white beans (any kind), cauliflower, onion, peeled and pressed garlic, cherry tomatoes each sliced in half, tomato paste, fresh parsley, cumin, smoked paprika, summer savory, and water almost to the fill line, seal, and cook for 1 hour and 30 minutes.

TAGINE VARIATION   To a pressure cooker, add dry white beans (any kind), a can of cooked white beans (any kind), cauliflower, orange bell pepper, cherry tomatoes each sliced in half, canned pumpkin, fresh cilantro, garam masala, dried ground ginger, dried sage, turmeric, and water almost to the fill line, seal, and cook for 1 hour and 30 minutes.

21. Blueberry Cobbler

These cobblers surround a whole grain biscuit with a sea of fruit concentrate. Two packages of frozen fruit and two cans of (unsweetened) frozen juice concentrate should see you through the week.

biscuit

¼ cup large-size whole grain like barley, brown rice, buckwheat groats, farro, kamut, spelt, rye, wheat, or triticale (two kinds are nice)
½ cup whole wheat flour
½ cup whole grain flour
¼ teaspoon (aluminum-free) baking powder
dash coarse salt
2 teaspoons oil

topping

a third of a 10-ounce package frozen blueberries
a third of a 12-ounce can frozen unsweetened apple juice concentrate (like Old Orchard's Apple Juice Concentrate)
½ teaspoon ground cinnamon

Toast some whole grains in a small saucepan on high heat until aromatic. Place foil sheet on foil tray, spray sheet with oil. Mix whole wheat flour, whole grain flour, (aluminum-free) baking powder, and coarse salt, add the whole grains which by now should be golden and aromatic, oil, and stir enough water to make a shapeable dough. Form into a rough bowl shape and place the batter (without stopping to knead it) onto the oil-sprayed foil on foil tray, bake at 350° 20 minutes until crust golden-brown. In the small saucepan place frozen blueberries, apple juice concentrate (like Old Orchard's Apple Juice Concentrate), and cinnamon, bring to boiling, turn off heat. Place baked biscuit in serving dish and add topping.

BERRY VARIATION Toast whole grain in a small saucepan on high heat until aromatic. Place foil sheet on foil tray, spray sheet with oil. Mix whole wheat flour, whole grain flour, (aluminum-free) baking powder, and coarse salt, add the whole grains which by now should be golden and aromatic, oil, and just enough water to make a shapeable dough. Form into a rough bowl shape and place the batter (without stopping to knead it) onto the oil-sprayed foil on foil tray, bake at 350° 20 minutes until crust golden-brown. In the small saucepan place raspberries or other frozen berry, unsweetened grape juice concentrate (like Old Orchard's Frozen Grape Juice Concentrate), agave nectar, and allspice, bring to boiling, turn off heat. Place baked biscuit in serving dish and add topping.

22. **Lentil Stew**

Stock adds depth to these nourishing stews of lentils, which can be brown, green, red, or black.

vegetable stock
4 carrots
4 stalks celery
1 onion
1 sweet potato
1 (15-ounce) can tomatoes
1 (8-ounce) package mushrooms
1 bunch fresh parsley
5 bay leaves
1 teaspoon allspice berries
1 teaspoon peppercorns

2½ cups (one 16-ounce package) dry lentils, any kind
4 carrots
4 stalks celery
1 onion
1 (15-ounce) can diced tomatoes
1 bunch fresh parsley
dash caraway seeds

Make a vegetable stock by coarsely chopping carrots, celery, onion, and sweet potato – no peeling or special care needed – adding canned diced tomatoes, fresh mushrooms, fresh parsley, bay leaves, allspice berries, and peppercorns into one large stockpot half-filled with water, boil for 30 minutes. To a pressure cooker add dry lentils (any kind), finely chopped carrots, celery, onion, canned diced tomatoes, fresh parsley, caraway seeds, and pour the vegetable stock through a drainer to add it as well up to the fill mark (save any excess stock to add after cooking), cover and seal the pressure cooker, and cook for 15 minutes.

PUMPKIN VARIATION   Make a corn stock by adding frozen corn and coarsely chopped carrots, celery, onion, turnip, fresh cilantro, canned diced tomatoes, fresh mushrooms, and peppercorns into one large stockpot half-filled with water, boil for 30 minutes. To a pressure cooker add dry lentils (any kind), finely chopped carrot, celery, onion, canned cooked pumpkin, canned diced tomatoes, a package of fresh watercress, and pour the corn stock through a drainer to add it as well up to the fill mark, cover and seal the pressure cooker (save any excess stock to add after cooking), and cook for 15 minutes.

23. Sweet Short-Grain Pancakes

These reinterpreted pancakes replace starchy refined flour with whole grain goodness. The sweetness referred to in the title is imparted by maple syrup, or, if you're feeling adventurous, a homemade syrup made from applesauce and apple juice concentrate.

1 tablespoon almonds, coarsely ground
½ cup whole wheat flour
½ cup whole grain flour
1 tablespoon small-size whole grain (like Whole Foods' Super Grains)
1 teaspoon (aluminum-free) baking powder
1 teaspoon coarse salt
½ teaspoon dried thyme

Over the weekend, coarsely grind almonds and refrigerate. When ready to make, mix whole wheat flour, whole grain flour, a small whole grain (like Whole Foods' Super Grains), some of the coarsely ground almonds, (aluminum-free) baking powder, coarse salt, dried thyme, and enough water to make a very pourable batter. Use less than a tablespoon of oil per pancake and keeping the pancakes small enough to flip easily, pour, fry on medium heat until edges crisp, flip, fry other side same amount of time, and repeat for each pancake, adding water to the mix if needed to keep it very pourable (but not so much water that the edges develop numerous holes in them when frying). Serve with maple syrup.

SUNFLOWER VARIATION   Mix whole grain flour, whole wheat flour, whole grain cereal, ground flaxseed, a small whole grain (like Whole Foods' Super Grains), sunflower kernels, (aluminum-free) baking powder, coarse salt, ground nutmeg, and enough water to make a very pourable batter. Using a frying pan and a small amount of oil, pour a pancake small enough to flip easily, fry each side on medium heat a few minutes until edges crisp, then flip and fry the other side. Add water to the mix if needed to keep it very pourable (but not so much water that the edges develop numerous holes in them when frying). Serve with maple syrup or try an exotic syrup like banana, blueberry, or pumpkin pie. Or make your own apple syrup in a medium-size soup pot, heating unsweetened apple juice concentrate, unsweetened applesauce, ground cinnamon, and ground cloves to a low boil about 10 minutes or until its volume is reduced by about half.

24. No-Egg Frittata

These omelets use nutritional yeast – a nutty, cheesy-tasting dairy alternative made from yeast, sugar cane, and beet molasses – and cubed protein-rich extra-firm tofu, and get a protein boost from pea protein, like Now Foods Pea Protein, a neutral-tasting powder that gets along well with nutritional yeast. Try marinated baked tofu, like Wildwood Organic SprouTofu. 3 (6-ounce) baked tofus, a (32-ounce) soy milk, along with an onion and 2 bell peppers (or 2 8-ounce packages of mushrooms and a 14-ounce can of tomatoes) should be enough for a week of these delicious dinner meals.

1 teaspoon oil
1 (4-ounce) section of baked tofu
2 tablespoons onion
2 tablespoons bell pepper, any color
1 tablespoon fresh parsley
1 scoop pea protein
2 teaspoons nutritional yeast
dash teaspoon coarse black pepper
dash dried tarragon
dash teaspoon turmeric
1 tablespoon unsweetened soy milk

In a frying pan, simmer oil, baked tofu, onion, bell pepper (any color), fresh parsley, pea protein, nutritional yeast, coarse black pepper, dried tarragon, turmeric, and unsweetened soy milk on medium heat a few minutes until slightly thickened. Serve hot.

TOMATO BASIL VARIATION   Before serving, use a frying pan to simmer oil, baked tofu, onion, mushrooms, a little pressed garlic, fresh arugula, canned diced tomatoes, pea protein, nutritional yeast, dried basil, smoked paprika, turmeric, and unsweetened soy milk on medium heat a few minutes until slightly thickened. Serve hot.

25. **Multigrain Bagels**

These whole-grain-based bagels go great with vegan cream cheese.

½ **tablespoon whole grain flour for coating**
½ **cup whole wheat flour**
½ **cup whole grain flour**
1 tablespoon ground flaxseed
1 tablespoon whole brown sugar (like Wholesome's Sucanat)
½ **teaspoon coarse salt**
oil
dried minced onion, sesame seeds, dried minced garlic, or poppy seeds

Bring water and dash of coarse salt to boil in a medium soup pot. Place foil sheet on foil tray, spray sheet with oil. Mix whole wheat flour, whole grain flour, ground flaxseed, whole sugar (like Wholesome's Sucanat), coarse salt, and enough water to make a dough. Shape the dough into two balls and drop them into the hot salted water. Once the water is boiling, turn off the heat, fish out each bagel using a hand-held sieve, drain it, and place onto a cutting board to cool. Then push your finger through each ball one at a time to make a bagel's characteristic torus shape, and place on the tray. Sprinkle bagel with either dried minced garlic, dried minced onion, poppy seeds, or sesame seeds, drip a small amount of oil over the topping, bake at 350° 20 minutes until golden and crispy. Top with a dollop of no-palm-oil vegan cream cheese (like Kite Hill's Plain Cream Cheese).

YEASTED VARIATION   Bring water to boil in a medium soup pot. Warm ⅓ cup of water in microwave 30 seconds and adjust until water very hot yet tolerable to finger immersion, add pinch of whole sugar (like Wholesome's Sucanat), a tablespoon of yeast, stir, and set aside set aside in a draft-free area for 15 minutes to proof. Place foil sheet on foil tray, spray sheet with oil. Mix whole wheat flour, whole grain flour, whole sugar, coarse salt, and the proofed yeast mixture to make a dough. Add a little baking soda to the boiling water. Shape the dough into two balls and drop them into the hot baking-soda-added water. Once the water is boiling, turn off the heat, fish out each bagel using a hand-held sieve, drain it, and place onto a cutting board to cool. Then push your finger through each ball one at a time to make a bagel's characteristic torus shape, and place on the tray. Sprinkle bagel with either dried minced garlic, dried minced onion, poppy seeds, or sesame seeds, drip a small amount of oil over the topping, bake at 350° 20 minutes until golden and crispy. Top with a dollop of no-palm-oil vegan cream cheese (like Kite Hill's Plain Cream Cheese).

26. Squash Stew

White beans combine with warm, comforting squash and the earthy flavor of dried mushrooms.

1 large squash
1 (15-ounce) can cooked white beans (any kind)
2½ cups (one 16-ounce package) dry white beans (any kind)
2 carrots
1 onion
1 (14.5-ounce) can diced tomatoes
1 (4-ounce package) dried mushrooms (any kind)
1 bunch fresh parsley
2 teaspoons dried ground ginger
2 teaspoons *herbes de Provence* seasoning

Slice squash in half and roast on foil on a foil tray at 350° for 1 hour and 30 minutes. To a pressure cooker add dry white beans (any kind), a can of cooked white beans (any kind), carrots, onion, canned diced tomatoes, dried mushrooms, fresh parsley, dried ground ginger, and *herbes de Provence* seasoning, fill with water only up to 3/4ths of the way to the maximum to leave some room for the squash. Seal and cook for 1 hour and 30 minutes. Remove baked squash from oven, scoop out and discard the seeds, scoop out the cooled cooked squash, place in a bowl, mush it thoroughly with your fingers and hands until it is soft with no lumps, add about same amount of water as there is squash, thoroughly mush that to mix it, and add it to the cooked stew and stir.

SUMMER (OR WINTER) VARIATION   For a taste of summer (or winter), slice squash in half and roast it on oil-sprayed foil at 350° for 1 hour and 30 minutes. To a pressure cooker add dry white beans (or kidney beans), onion, peeled and pressed garlic, a can of cooked white beans (or dark beans), frozen green peas, mushrooms, tomatoes (or tomatoes, tomato paste, soy sauce, and ketchup), dried mushrooms (or fake steak like Eat Meati's Mushroom Root Protein Carne Asada Steaks) and summer savory (or dried thyme), fill with water only up to 3/4ths of the way to the maximum to leave some room for the squash. Seal and cook for 1 hour and 30 minutes. Remove baked squash from oven, scoop out and discard the seeds, scoop out the cooled cooked squash, place in a bowl, mush it thoroughly with your fingers and hands until it is soft with no lumps, add about same amount of water as there is squash, thoroughly mush that to mix it, and add it to the cooked stew and stir.

27. Around-the-World Grains

Go around the world without leaving the pantry with these grain dishes made from staples you keep on hand. Small grains like amaranth, millet, quinoa, short-grain rice, and teff turn tender with as little as 5 minutes in the pressure cooker, while larger, tougher grains like whole buckwheat groats, hulled rye, sorghum, spelt, or wheat berries can take as long as an hour but yield a complex nutty flavor that is worth the wait. If you're in a hurry, bring a covered medium soup pot to boil, add whole grain pasta, cover, turn off the heat, wait 15 minutes, and add any of the seasonings below. Occasionally, try substituting the fresh form of one or more of the dry seasoning ingredients.

½ cup whole grain

seasoning
1 teaspoon extra virgin olive oil
¼ teaspoon coarse salt

Place the whole grain in a pressure cooker, add twice as much water as grain, seal, and cook 5 to 60 minutes, until tender but not mushy (the larger the grain, the longer the cooking). Drain and try a California blend of dried cilantro, dried tarragon, dried thyme, oil, and salt; the French *herbes de Provence* of marjoram, oregano, rosemary, savory, and thyme, extra virgin olive oil, and salt; the Parisian *quatre épices* of the slightest hint of cloves, dried ground ginger, nutmeg, black pepper, oil, and salt; or a Spanish *condimento* of coriander, smoked paprika, saffron, extra virgin olive oil, and salt.

AROUND-THE-WORLD VARIATION   Place the whole grain in a pressure cooker, add twice as much water as grain, seal, and cook 5 to 60 minutes, until tender but not mushy (the larger the grain, the longer the cooking). Drain and continue around the world with an Italian *stagionatura* of dried garlic granules, a pinch of dried oregano, dried parsley, and dried sage, extra virgin olive oil, and salt; the Lebanese seven spices of allspice, black pepper, cinnamon, ground cloves, coriander, cumin, and nutmeg (or just use a premade mixture), extra virgin olive oil, and salt; an Indian *masala* of *garam masala*, oil, and salt; or a Samoan *fa'ama'i* of toasted sesame oil, soy sauce, sesame seed, whole sugar, and dry seaweed toasted briefly over an open flame and crumbled.

28. "Steak" and "Fries"

For this week, have these "steaks" or "gyros" made from protein-rich seitan with baked potato "fries" for lunch, and for supper, make a simple chili of dry beans, canned beans, onion, carrots, green pepper, canned diced tomatoes, fresh parsley, a jar of mild salsa, and enough water to fill the pressure cooker almost full, seal and cook for 1 hour and 30 minutes.

steak

2 tablespoons wheat gluten (like Bob's Red Mill Gluten Flour)
2 tablespoons bean flour
shoyu or tamari soy sauce for dipping
ketchup for dipping

fries

1-3 Russet, red, yellow, white, purple, fingerling, or petite potatoes
oil
(no-sugar-added) bread crumbs (like Whole Foods Plain Bread Crumbs)
smoked paprika
coarse salt

Place foil sheet on foil tray, spray sheet with oil. Cut a potato or two into bite-size chunks, place in a plastic bag, add some oil, coarse salt, smoked paprika, (no-sugar-added) bread crumbs (like Whole Foods Plain Bread Crumbs), shake, place the breaded potatoes on oil-sprayed foil on foil tray, roast 350° 45 minutes or until crispy but not burnt. Put some soy sauce in one bowl and some ketchup in another. Make steaks bites by combining equal parts wheat gluten flour (like Bob's Red Mill Gluten Flour) and bean flour and just enough water to form 5-8 bite-size pieces, dip in the soy sauce, the ketchup, then fry with oil on medium heat a few minutes each side to lightly brown. Serve the "steaks" with potato "fries."

"GYRO" VARIATION Place foil sheet on foil tray, spray sheet with oil. Cut a potato or two into bite-size chunks, place in a plastic bag, add some oil, coarse salt, dried dill, (no-sugar-added) bread crumbs (like Whole Foods Plain Bread Crumbs), shake, place the breaded potatoes on oil-sprayed foil on foil tray, roast 350° 45 minutes or until crispy but not burnt. Put some soy sauce in one bowl and some mustard in another. Make steaks bites by combining equal parts wheat gluten flour (like Bob's Red Mill Gluten Flour) and bean flour and just enough water to form 5-8 bite-size pieces, dip in the soy sauce, the mustard, then fry with oil on medium heat a few minutes each side, adding sliced onion, sliced collard greens, stirring and flipping until everything lightly browned. Warm one or two whole grain pitas in oven (put them on the tray with the potatoes for 5 minutes), layer pitas with steak bites, the sauteed pieces-onion-greens mixture, thin slices of fresh tomato, vegan yogurt (like Daiya's Greek Yogurt Alternative), fold, and serve. Serve the "gyros" with potato "fries."

29. Sun-Dried Tomato Polenta

We end the bean-grain pairings with this festive lunchtime polenta, which, if you've been following along with these recipes, finishes out three months of cooking. For supper this week, take a break from making a bean-based stew and just mix beans with store-bought single-serving soup (accompanied by whole grain snacks, fresh salad, peanut butter, and an apple).

stuffing
1 teaspoon oil
¼ cup onion, diced
2 garlic cloves, minced or pressed
¼ cup Swiss chard
¼ cup sun-dried tomatoes, sliced
¼ cup croutons

polenta
¾ cup coarse corn meal

In a medium soup pot, simmer oil, onion, garlic, and Swiss chard on medium heat until onion translucent, about 5 minutes. Add corn meal and just enough water to make a thick but stirrable polenta, using a water-to-corn-meal ratio of about 1:1, stirring occasionally. Once the polenta is thick enough to hold its shape, turn off heat, add some sun-dried tomatoes and croutons, stir again once, scoop everything out, place on the tray, sprinkle on a little salt, and bake at 350° 20 minutes until crust golden crisp.

CHESTNUT CRANBERRY VARIATION   Cut an "X" into a few chestnuts, roast 400° for 20 minutes on oil-sprayed foil on a foil tray, turn off heat; if using other nuts, roast 5 minutes. In a medium soup pot, simmer oil, onion, fresh parsley, dried sage, and brandy (optional) on low heat until onion translucent, about 5 minutes. Peel and skin the cooled chestnuts. Add corn meal and just enough water to make a thick but stirrable polenta, using a water-to-corn-meal mixture of about 1:1, stirring occasionally. Once the polenta is thick enough to hold its shape, turn off heat, add some cranberries (or other in-season pitless berry), croutons, and the skinned and peeled roasted chestnuts or nuts, stir again once, scoop everything out, place on the tray, sprinkle on a little salt, and bake at 350° 20 minutes until crust golden crisp.

30. **Berry-Nut Cookies**

Finish each three-month cycle of food with these celebratory cookies. Whole sugar – like dark muscovado, demerara, or turbinado – is still sugar, but at least has more flavor and nutrients. Next week, start back again with Minestrone (#6, page 96) and Cornmeal-Crusted Soy Steak Sandwiches (#7, page 97).

1 cup whole wheat flour
1 cup whole grain flour
½ cup whole sugar (like Wholesome's Sucanat)
1 tablespoon ground flaxseed
1 teaspoon (aluminum-free) baking powder
½ teaspoon coarse salt
½ pint fresh seedless/pitless berry
½ cup mixed nuts
½ cup oil
¼ cup maple syrup (or agave nectar)
2 teaspoons vanilla extract
½ cup water

Place each of two foil sheets on to two foil trays (you'll two fit the cookies without crowding), spray each sheet with oil. Mix whole wheat flour, whole grain flour, whole sugar (like Wholesome's Sucanat), ground flaxseed, (aluminum-free) baking powder, coarse salt, the (seedless/pitless) berries, mixed nuts, oil, maple syrup (or agave nectar), vanilla extract, and just enough water to make a wet but sticky dough. Place tablespoon-sized dollops onto the oil-sprayed foil. Bake cookies at 350° 20 minutes only until tops golden but the dough, which will solidify more as it cools, still soft. Refrigerate.

MOCHA CHOCOLATE CHIP VARIATION   Place each of two foil sheets on to two foil trays and spray each sheet with oil. Mix whole wheat flour, whole grain flour, whole sugar (like Wholesome's Sucanat), ground coffee beans, ground flaxseed, (aluminum-free) baking powder, coarse salt, then add vegan chocolate chips, oil, maple syrup (or agave nectar), coffee liqueur (like Kahlúa), vanilla extract, and just enough water to make a wet but sticky dough, mix again, and place tablespoon-sized dollops onto the oil-sprayed foil. Bake cookies at 350° 20 minutes only until tops golden but the dough, which will solidify more as it cools, still soft. Refrigerate.

Section 5

CONTINUING ON

ndividualized, self-directed exercise has been the focus of this book, but fitness can also be pursued as a group effort. Working out with a partner, joining a gym or health club, and playing sports can all add a thrill to pursuing fitness. While I have emphasized body-weight strengthening and jogging for their simplicity, ease of access, and effectiveness, alternatives like bicycling, swimming, cardiovascular kickboxing, and martial arts each provide their own unique benefits. If you're a group person, organized sports and fitness, no longer the exclusive province of the young athlete, are becoming available for an ever-greater variety of individuals. Every year new gyms and health clubs open to provide a wider range of pleasant environments for exercise. Indeed, there is considerable evidence to show that resistance training with weights may offer even more gains in strength and body composition than calisthenics alone. Over time, you might find the gym – with its variety of machines, free weights, and aerobic equipment – to be worthy sanctuary for practicing higher-intensity training. Each exercise in this book has its parallel in free weights and exercise equipment.

Most workouts take up an hour or less of your day. What you do during the rest of your time can powerfully reinforce a workout's effects – or almost completely undo them.

- *Make it happen.* Solidify your fitness habit by making an appointment for your workout and treating it just like any other important commitment. Once in a while, use a notepad to record what you've done.

- *Do what you like.* The best exercise is the kind you enjoy. A workout is a tool for concentrating a day's worth of exercise into a short time period; physical activities like sports, carpentry, yard work, or hiking spread exercise out into longer periods of activity you really enjoy, and can refreshingly counterbalance the structured nature of workouts. Out of all the activities you enjoy, identify those that require the greatest physical effort, and spend more time doing them. Thanks to the enormous magnifying power of time, even simple activities have a deep effect over a lifetime when repeated: over just one year, for example, new dog owners lost 14 pounds simply by walking their dogs.[383]

- *Walk.* Get things done and help your body at the same time by choosing to walk. Make walking a social activity and include your kids, dog, family, and friends, who might enjoy the exercise along with you. Keep a pair of walking or running shoes in your desk at work. A walking break will energize you better than a coffee break. Walk part of your commute, after lunch, to the store, to social events, or to your place of worship. Park farther away from buildings, or take the stairs instead of the escalator. Find scenic places to walk and visit them; become a tourist in your own city. Over a lifetime, the minutes you spend walking add up to big health benefits.

- *Inculcate better TV habits.* Confirming the obvious, studies show heavy television viewing leads to heavy viewers. In the average American home, the TV is on for some seven hours every day.[384] Turn off your TV for a day, a week, or more, and check out tvturnoff.org for more ideas and inspiration. Or at least replace habitual hours of dull TV with fewer minutes of more interesting programming. New services and technology like Netflix and TiVo, by giving you greater control over what you watch and when, can, if you make up your mind to do it, shrink your total television watching time by exchanging dull, habitual watching for rarer but more exciting viewing experiences. Even children who reduced TV viewing to only one hour a day gained, in over just the relatively brief nine-month period of the study, an average two pounds less in fat than their peers.[385]

■ *Get into cooking.* Follow a routine of making a grocery list based on recipes for healthy meals that you will like, going to the food store at least once a week to get fresh food, and regularly cooking it up, some items fresh for each meal, others, as time dictates, in larger batches to last the week, and get your family and the people in your life to cook with you.

With the experience and skill you'll gain from practicing these workouts and recipes, you will be ready for a future that will be a great time for learning about exercise, nutrition, and fitness. Even now, there is an galaxy of great fitness books out there. Before leaving you with a bookshelf's worth of some of my favorites, along with a choice line from each, I want to thank you for taking the time to read this book. If you feel so inclined, I'd love to hear from you how the advice in this book worked out for you. I want to hear what worked for you, in the exercise advice, the workouts, the nutrition advice, and the recipes – and also what didn't. I'm also interested in your ideas on how to make this book better in ways that preserve its simplicity. If you notice any typos or grammatical errors, I'd appreciate hearing about those, too. Finally, if you'd like a copy of the routines, the recipes, or the references (including in a linked form so you can click on any of the underlined references to see its abstract online at the United States National Library of Medicine at the National Institutes of Health website, pubmed.gov), I'd be happy to provide you with any of those. You can contact me at pgrohne@yahoo.com. I hope this book helps you enjoy good health and a full life!

A BOOKSHELF'S WORTH: 15 HEALTHFUL BOOKS

AUTHOR	TITLE	SUBLIME PASSAGE
Elaine Marieb	*Human Anatomy & Physiology*	"You are only as old as your arteries." - page 659
William McArdle, Frank Katch, and Victor Katch	*Exercise Physiology*	"Physical fitness protects against death." - page 958
Stew Smith	*The Complete Guide to Navy SEAL Fitness*	"You can do anything you set your mind to." - page 16
Daniel Goleman	*Working With Emotional Intelligence*	"Mistakes are treasures, a chance to improve." - page 127
Jack Heggie	*Running With the Whole Body*	"The next time you run, start off slowly and feel your feet coming down onto the ground." - page 130
Lam Kam Chuen	*Step-by-Step Tai Chi*	"On the outside you are moving; on the inside you are still." - page 67
John Scott	*Ashtanga Yoga*	"Initially this pose can feel very difficult, but as you grow more familiar with it, it can become a place of solace and tranquility." - page 74

Steve Tarpinian	*The Essential Swimmer*	"Because we evolved from fish (did you know human enbryos still have gills?), we have great potential for being comfortable in the water." - page 1
Patrick McKeown	*The Oxygen Advantage*	"If you reduce your breathing, you will teach your body to breathe more efficiently, and you will become healthier." - page 7
Walter Willett	*Eat, Drink, and Be Healthy*	"Few of us take advantage of the incredible bounty of fruits and vegetables grown in this country and elsewhere." - page 118
Eric Schlosser	*Fast Food Nation*	"The cattle now packed into feedlots get little exercise and live amid pools of manure. 'You shouldn't eat dirty food and dirty water,' the official told me. 'But we still think we can give animals dirty food and dirty water.'" - page 190
Howard Lyman and Glen Merzer	*Mad Cowboy*	"An insidious spiral develops: overgrazing leads to more dust and drier air (as less water transpires from vegetation), leading to less rain, resulting in still less plant life." - page 147
Robin Robertson	*Vegan Planet*	"Chestnuts have a fair amount of protein and are a good source of calcium, potassium, B complex vitamins, magnesium, and iron. To cook chestnuts, pierce the shells with a sharp knife, cutting an X in the shell. Then boil or roast them at 375° and peel them while still fairly hot, using a sharp knife to remove the outer shell and the inner skin." - page 413
Isa Chandra Moskowitz and Terry Hope Romero	*Veganomicon*	"Way back in the '80s when people thought that 'mousse for hair' was a good idea, fat of all kinds became the cold-war level threat to the country." - page 22
Janet Gronnow	*15-Minute Vegan Meals*	"Your senses will be a great way to keep tabs on your cooking is going." - page 11

References

Behind the advice I give are citations referencing relevant research. If a citation is underlined, it means that the full summary, or abstract, is available online at the United States Library of Medicine's publicly accessible database, PubMed, at pubmed.gov.

1 Little JP, Safdar A, Benton CR, Wright DC. Skeletal muscle and beyond: the role of exercise as a mediator of systemic mitochondrial biogenesis. Appl Physiol Nutr Metab. 2011 Oct;36(5):598-607

2 Pigozzi F, Rizzo M, Giombini A, Parisi A, Fagnani F, Borrione P. Bone mineral density and sport: effect of physical activity. J Sports Med Phys Fitness. 2009 Jun;49(2):177-8

3 Leung FP, Yung LM, Laher I, Yao X, Chen ZY, Huang Y. Exercise, vascular wall and cardiovascular diseases: an update (Part 1). Sports Med. 2008;38(12):1009-24

4 Langberg H, Skovgaard D, Petersen LJ, Bulow J, Kjaer M. Type I collagen synthesis and degradation in peritendinous tissue after exercise determined by microdialysis in humans. J Physiol. 1999 Nov 15;521 Pt 1:299-306

5 Alves CR, Tessaro VH, Teixeira LA, Murakava K, Roschel H, Gualano B, Takito MY. Influence of acute high-intensity aerobic interval exercise bout on selective attention and short-term memory tasks. Percept Mot Skills. 2014 Feb;118(1):63-72

6 Hughes JR. Psychological effects of habitual aerobic exercise: a critical review. Prev Med. 1984 Jan;13(1):66-78

7 Kovács E, Sztruhár Jónásné I, Karóczi CK, Korpos A, Gondos T. Effects of a multimodal exercise program on balance, functional mobility and fall risk in older adults with cognitive impairment: a randomized controlled single-blind study. Eur J Phys Rehabil Med. 2013 Oct;49(5):639--48

8 Gremeaux V, Gayda M, Lepers R, Sosner P, Juneau M, Nigam A. Exercise and longevity. Maturitas. 2012 Dec;73(4):312-7

9 Alter DA, Wijeysundera HC, Franklin B, Austin PC, Chong A, Oh PI, Tu JV, Stukel TA. Obesity, lifestyle risk-factors, and health service outcomes among healthy middle-aged adults in Canada. BMC Health Serv Res. 2012 Aug 4;12:238

10 Sobngwi E, Mbanya JC, Unwin NC, Kengne AP, Fezeu L, Minkoulou EM, Aspray TJ, Alberti KG. Physical activity and its relationship with obesity, hypertension and diabetes in urban and rural Cameroon. Int J Obes Relat Metab Disord. 2002 Jul;26(7):1009-16

11 Kartono A. Modified minimal model for effect of physical exercise on insulin sensitivity and glucose effectiveness in type 2 diabetes and healthy human. Theory Biosci. 2013 Sep;132(3):195-206

12 Willis FB, Smith FM, Willis AP. Frequency of exercise for body fat loss: a controlled, cohort study. J Strength Cond Res. 2009 Nov;23(8):2377-80

13 American Academy of Family Physicians. The exercise habit. Created January, 1996, updated December, 2009

14 National Center for Health Statistics, press release April 6, 2010, http://www.cdc.gov/nchs/data/hestat/physicalactivity/physicalactivity.htm

15 Health and Social Care Information Centre. Statistics on obesity, physical activity and diet: England, January 2008. http://www.ic.nhs.uk/pubs/opadjan08

16 International Health, Racquet, and Sportsclub Association, press release March 31, 2010, http://cms.ihrsa.org/index.cfm?fuseaction=page.viewPage&pageID=21108

17 Willardson JM. The effectiveness of resistance exercises performed on unstable equipment. Strength and Conditioning Journal, 2004;5:70-74

18 Pollock ML, Gettman LR, Milesis CA, Bah MD, Durstine L, Johnson RB. Effect of frequency and duration of

training on attrition and incidence of injury. Medicine & Science in Sports and Exercise, 1977;9:31-36

[19] Ballor DL, Keesey RE. A meta-analysis of the factors affecting exercise-induced changes in body mass, fat mass and fat-free mass in males and females. Int J Obes. 1991 Nov;15(11):717-26

[20] Buchowski MS, Townsend KM, Chen KY, Acra SA, Sun M. Energy expenditure determined by self-reported physical activity is related to body fatness. Obes Res. 1999 Jan;7(1):23-33

[21] Tremblay A, Despres JP, Bouchard C. The effects of exercise-training on energy balance and adipose tissue morphology and metabolism. Sports Med. 1985 May-Jun;2(3):223-33

[22] LaMonte MJ, Durstine JL, Addy CL, Irwin ML, Ainsworth BE. Physical activity, physical fitness, and Framingham 10-year risk score: the cross-cultural activity participation study. J Cardiopulm Rehabil. 2001 Mar-Apr;21(2):63-70

[23] Martinez DG, Nicolau JC, Lage RL, Toschi-Dias E, de Matos LD, Alves MJ, Trombetta IC, Dias da Silva VJ, Middlekauff HR, Negrão CE, Rondon MU. Effects of long-term exercise training on autonomic control in myocardial infarction patients. Hypertension. 2011 Dec;58(6):1049-56

[24] Downing J, Balady GJ. The role of exercise training in heart failure. J Am Coll Cardiol. 2011 Aug 2;58(6):561-9

[25] Huebschmann AG, Kohrt WM, Regensteiner JG. Exercise attenuates the premature cardiovascular aging effects of type 2 diabetes mellitus. Vasc Med. 2011 Oct;16(5):378-90

[26] Minor MA. Exercise in the treatment of osteoarthritis. Rheum Dis Clin North Am. 1999 May;25(2):397-415, viii

[27] Wolff E, Gaudlitz K, von Lindenberger BL, Plag J, Heinz A, Ströhle A. Exercise and physical activity in mental disorders. Eur Arch Psychiatry Clin Neurosci. 2011 Nov;261 Suppl 2:S186-91

[28] Allen J, Morelli V. Aging and exercise. Clin Geriatr Med. 2011 Nov;27(4):661-71

[29] Carlisle D. Better than any drug. Nurs Stand. 2012 Jan 18-24;26(20):18-9.

[30] Anderson JW, Konz EC, Frederich RC, Wood CL. Long-term weight-loss maintenance: a meta-analysis of US studies. Am J Clin Nutr. 2001 Nov;74(5):579-84

[31] Harvard Medical School, September, 2005. http://www.health.harvard.edu/newsweek/The_quickie_workout.htm

[32] Kraemer WJ, Fleck SJ, Evans WJ. Strength and power training: physiological mechanisms of adaptation. Exerc Sport Sci Rev. 1996;24:363-97

[33] Sale DG. Neural adaptation to resistance training. Med Sci Sports Exerc. 1988 Oct;20(5 Suppl):S135-45

[34] Matoba H, Gollnick PD. Response of skeletal muscle to training. Sports Med. 1984 May-Jun;1(3):240-51

[35] Expert panel: executive summary of the clinical guidelines on the identification, evaluation, and treatment of overweight and obesity in adults. Arch Intern Med 1998;158:1855-1867

[36] Schjerve IE, Tyldum GA, Tjønna AE, Stølen T, Loennechen JP, Hansen HE, Haram PM, Heinrich G, Bye A, Najjar SM, Smith GL, Slørdahl SA, Kemi OJ, Wisløff U. Both aerobic endurance and strength training programmes improve cardiovascular health in obese adults. Clin Sci (Lond). 2008 Nov;115(9):283-93

[37] Lexell J, Taylor CC. Variability in muscle fibre areas in whole human quadriceps muscle: effects of increasing age. J Anat. 1991 Feb;174:239-49

[38] Klein CS, Rice CL, Marsh GD. Normalized force, activation, and coactivation in the arm muscles of young and old men. J Appl Physiol. 2001 Sep;91(3):1341-9

[39] Pleis JR, Lucas JW. Summary health statistics for U.S. adults: National Health Interview Survey, 2007. National Center for Health Statistics. Vital Health Stat 10(240). 2009. http://www.cdc.gov/nchs/nhis/physical_activity/pa_statistics.htm

[40] Wang Z, Ying Z, Bosy-Westphal A, Zhang J, Heller M, Later W, Heymsfield SB, Müller MJ. Evaluation of specific metabolic rates of major organs and tissues: comparison between men and women. Am J Hum Biol. 2011 May-Jun;23(3):333-8

[41] Wang Z, Heshka S, Gallagher D, Boozer CN, Kotler DP, Heymsfield SB. Resting energy expenditure-fat-free

mass relationship: new insights provided by body composition modeling. Am J Physiol Endocrinol Metab. 2000 Sep;279(3):E539-45

42 Withers RT, Sherman WM, Miller JM, Costill DL. Specificity of the anaerobic threshold in endurance trained cyclists and runners. Eur J Appl Physiol Occup Physiol. 1981;47(1):93-104

43 Reilly T, Morris T, Whyte G. The specificity of training prescription and physiological assessment: a review. J Sports Sci. 2009 Apr;27(6):575-89

44 Folland JP, Williams AG. The adaptations to strength training: morphological and neurological contributions to increased strength. Sports Med. 2007;37(2):145-68

45 Daub WB, Green HJ, Houston ME, Thomson JA, Fraser IG, Ranney DA. Specificity of physiologic adaptations resulting from ice-hockey training. Med Sci Sports Exerc. 1983;15(4):290-4

46 Gwinup G, Chelvam R, Steinberg T. Thickness of subcutaneous fat and activity of underlying muscles. Annals of Internal Medicine, 1971: 408-11

47 Vispute SS, Smith JD, Lecheminant JD, Hurley KS. The effect of abdominal exercise on abdominal fat. J Strength Cond Res. 2011 Sep;25(9):2559-64

48 Augustsson J, Esko A, Thomee R, Svantesson U. Weight training of the thigh muscles using closed vs. open chain exercises: a comparison of performance enhancement. Journal of Orthopedic Sports Physical Therapy. 1998 Jan;27(1):3-8

49 Blackburn JR, Morrissey MC. The relationship between open and closed kinetic chain strength of the lower limb and jumping performance. J Orthop Sports Phys Ther. 1998 Jun;27(6):430-5

50 Mazess RB. On aging bone loss. Clin Orthop. Clin Orthop. 1982 May;(165):239-52

51 World Health Organization, press release "Aging and Osteoporosis" April 7, 1999

52 Melton LJ 3rd. The prevalence of osteoporosis: gender and racial comparison. Calcif Tissue Int. 2001 Oct;69(4):179-81

53 González-Zabaleta J, Pita-Fernandez S, Seoane-Pillado T, López-Calviño B, Gonzalez-Zabaleta JL. Comorbidity as a predictor of mortality and mobility after hip fracture. Geriatr Gerontol Int. 2015 May 15

54 Kemmler W, Lauber D, Weineck J, Hensen J, Kalender W, Engelke K. Benefits of 2 Years of Intense Exercise on Bone Density, Physical Fitness, and Blood Lipids in Early Postmenopausal Osteopenic Women: Results of the Erlangen Fitness Osteoporosis Prevention Study (EFOPS). Arch Intern Med. 2004 May 24;164(10):1084-1091

55 Krolner B, Toft B. Vertebral bone loss: an unheeded side effect of therapeutic bed rest. Clinical Science (London). 1983 May;64(5):537-40

56 Issekutz B, Blizzrad JJ, Birkhead NC, Rodahl K. Effect of prolonged bed rest on urinary calcium output. J. Appl. Physiol. 1966;21(3):1013-1020

57 Skerry TM. The response of bone to mechanical loading and disuse: fundamental principles and influences on osteoblast/osteocyte homeostasis. Arch Biochem Biophys. 2008 May 15;473(2):117-23

58 Arkill KP, Winlove CP. Solute transport in the deep and calcified zones of articular cartilage. Osteoarthritis Cartilage. 2008 Jun;16(6):708-14; Quinn TM, Morel V, Meister JJ. Static compression of articular cartilage can reduce solute diffusivity and partitioning: implications for the chondrocyte biological response. J Biomech. 2001 Nov;34(11):1463-9

59 Urban JP. The chondrocyte: a cell under pressure. The chondrocyte: a cell under pressure. Br J Rheumatol. 1994 Oct;33(10):901-8

60 Carter DR, Wong M. Modelling cartilage mechanobiology. Philos Trans R Soc Lond B Biol Sci. 2003 Sep 29;358(1437):1461-71; Saadat E, Lan H, Majumdar S, Rempel DM, King KB. Long-term cyclical in vivo loading increases cartilage proteoglycan content in a spatially specific manner: an infrared microspectroscopic imaging and polarized light microscopy study. Arthritis Res Ther. 2006;8(5):R147

[61] Eckstein F, Hudelmaier M, Putz R. The effects of exercise on human articular cartilage. J Anat. 2006 Apr;208(4):491-512; Carter DR, Beaupré GS, Wong M, Smith RL, Andriacchi TP, Schurman DJ. The mechanobiology of articular cartilage development and degeneration. Clin Orthop Relat Res. 2004 Oct;(427 Suppl):S69-77

[62] Mcardle WD, Katch FI, Katch VL. Essentials of exercise physiology. Philadelphia: Lea & Febiger, 1994, p. 165

[63] Hillman CH, Erickson KI, Kramer AF. Be smart, exercise your heart: exercise effects on brain and cognition. Nat Rev Neurosci. 2008 Jan;9(1):58-65

[64] Pal S, Radavelli-Bagatini S, Ho S. Potential benefits of exercise on blood pressure and vascular function. J Am Soc Hypertens. 2013 Nov-Dec;7(6):494-506

[65] Roberts CK, Hevener AL, Barnard RJ. Metabolic syndrome and insulin resistance: underlying causes and modification by exercise training. Compr Physiol. 2013 Jan;3(1):1-58

[66] Hoffman MD, Hoffman DR. Exercisers achieve greater acute exercise-induced mood enhancement than nonexercisers. Arch Phys Med Rehabil. 2008 Feb;89(2):358-63

[67] Puterman E, O'Donovan A, Adler NE, Tomiyama AJ, Kemeny M, Wolkowitz OM, Epel E. Physical activity moderates effects of stressor-induced rumination on cortisol reactivity. Psychosom Med. 2011 Sep;73(7):604-11

[68] Daniels J. Obesity: America's epidemic. Am J Nurs. 2006 Jan;106(1):40-9

[69] Fields LE, Burt VL, Cutler JA, Hughes J, Roccella EJ, Sorlie P. The burden of adult hypertension in the United States 1999 to 2000: a rising tide. Hypertension. 2004 Oct;44(4):398-404

[70] Tesauro M, Cardillo C. Obesity, blood vessels and metabolic syndrome. Acta Physiol (Oxf). 2011 Sep;203(1):279-86

[71] Bogaert YE, Schrier RW. Into the future: prevention of diabetes. Contrib Nephrol. 2011;170:256-63

[72] Roemmich JN, Lambiase MJ, Balantekin KN, Feda DM, Dorn J. Stress, behavior, and biology: risk factors for cardiovascular diseases in youth. Exerc Sport Sci Rev. 2014 Oct;42(4):145-52

[73] Najafian J, Mohammadifard N, Naeini FF, Nouri F. Relation between usual daily walking time and metabolic syndrome. Niger Med J. 2014 Jan;55(1):29-33

[74] Charansonney OL. Physical activity and aging: a life-long story. Discov Med. 2011 Sep;12(64):177-85

[75] McArdle WD, Katch FI, Katch VL. Chapter 10, Energy expenditure during walking, jogging, running, and swimming, in Exercise physiology: energy, nutrition, and human performance, 5th ed., Baltimore, Maryland: Lippincott Williams & Wilkins, 2001, page 204

[76] McArdle WD, Katch FI, Katch VL. Chapter 10, Energy expenditure during walking, jogging, running, and swimming, in Exercise physiology: energy, nutrition, and human performance, 5th ed., Baltimore, Maryland: Lippincott Williams & Wilkins, 2001, page 209

[77] Wilkin LD, Cheryl A, Haddock BL. Energy expenditure comparison between walking and running in average fitness individuals. J Strength Cond Res. 2012 Apr;26(4):1039-44

[78] Cymet TC, Sinkov V. Does long-distance running cause osteoarthritis? J Am Osteopath Assoc. 2006 Jun;106(6):342-5

[79] Walther M, Kirschner S. [Is running associated with premature degenerative arthritis of the hip? A systematic review] Z Orthop Ihre Grenzgeb. 2004 Mar-Apr;142(2):213-20; Chakravarty EF, Hubert HB, Lingala VB, Zatarain E, Fries JF. Long distance running and knee osteoarthritis. A prospective study. Am J Prev Med. 2008 Aug;35(2):133-8

[80] Bruce B, Fries JF, Lubeck DP. Aerobic exercise and its impact on musculoskeletal pain in older adults: a 14 year prospective, longitudinal study. Arthritis Res Ther. 2005;7(6):R1263-70

[81] Fries JF, Singh G, Morfeld D, O'Driscoll P, Hubert H. Relationship of running to musculoskeletal pain with age. A six-year longitudinal study. Arthritis Rheum. 1996 Jan;39(1):64-72

[82] Rogers LQ, Macera CA, Hootman JM, Ainsworth BE, Blairi SN. The association between joint stress from

physical activity and self-reported osteoarthritis: an analysis of the Cooper Clinic data. Osteoarthritis Cartilage. 2002 Aug;10(8):617-22

83 Dunlop DD, Semanik P, Song J, Manheim LM, Shih V, Chang RW. Risk factors for functional decline in older adults with arthritis. Arthritis Rheum. 2005 Apr;52(4):1274-82

84 Schnohr P, Parner J, Lange P. [Joggers live longer. The Osterbro study, Article in Danish] Ugeskr Laeger. 2001 May 7;163(19):2633-5

85 Boutcher SH. High-intensity intermittent exercise and fat loss. J Obes. 2011;2011:868305

86 Ghosh AK. Anaerobic threshold: its concept and role in endurance sport. Malays J Med Sci. 2004 Jan;11(1):24-36

87 Mueller MJ, Maluf KS. Tissue adaptation to physical stress: a proposed "Physical Stress Theory" to guide physical therapist practice, education, and research. Phys Ther. 2002 Apr;82(4):383-403

88 Proske U, Morgan DL. Muscle damage from eccentric exercise: mechanism, mechanical signs, adaptation and clinical applications. J Physiol. 2001 Dec 1;537(Pt 2):333-45

89 Egan B, Zierath JR. Exercise metabolism and the molecular regulation of skeletal muscle adaptation. Cell Metab. 2013 Feb 5;17(2):162-84

90 Paton CD, Hopkins WG. Combining explosive and high-resistance training improves performance in competitive cyclists. J Strength Cond Res. 2005 Nov;19(4):826-30

91 Todd JS, Shurley JP, Todd TC. Thomas L. DeLorme and the science of progressive resistance exercise. J Strength Cond Res. 2012 Nov;26(11):2913-23

92 Glass SC, Stanton DR. Self-selected resistance training intensity in novice weightlifters. J Strength Cond Res. 2004 May;18(2):324-7

93 Krustrup P, Ferguson RA, Kjaer M, Bangsbo J. ATP and heat production in human skeletal muscle during dynamic exercise: higher efficiency of anaerobic than aerobic ATP resynthesis. J Physiol. 2003 May 15;549(Pt 1):255-69

94 Buist I, Bredeweg SW, van Mechelen W, Lemmink KA, Pepping GJ, Diercks RL. No effect of a graded training program on the number of running-related injuries in novice runners: a randomized controlled trial. Am J Sports Med. 2008 Jan;36(1):33-9

95 Rogind H, Bibow-Nielsen B, Jensen B, Moller HC, Frimodt-Moller H, Bliddal H. The effects of a physical training program on patients with osteoarthritis of the knees. Arch Phys Med Rehabil. 1998 Nov;79(11):1421-7

96 Vignon E, Valat JP, Rossignol M, Avouac B, Rozenberg S, Thoumie P, Avouac J, Nordin M, Hilliquin P. Osteoarthritis of the knee and hip and activity: a systematic international review and synthesis (OASIS). Joint Bone Spine. 2006 Jul;73(4):442-55

97 Delorme T, Watkins A: Techniques of progressive resistive exercise. Arch Phys Med Rehabil 29:263, 1948

98 Bellew JW, Yates JW, Gater DR. The initial effects of low-volume strength training on balance in untrained older men and women. J Strength Cond Res. 2003 Feb;17(1):121-8

99 Rhea MR. Determining the magnitude of treatment effects in strength training research through the use of the effect size. J Strength Cond Res. 2004 Nov;18(4):918-20

100 Kraemer WJ, Adams K, Cafarelli E, Dudley GA, Dooly C, Feigenbaum MS, Fleck SJ, Franklin B, Fry AC, Hoffman JR, Newton RU, Potteiger J, Stone MH, Ratamess NA, Triplett-McBride T; American College of Sports Medicine. American College of Sports Medicine position stand. Progression models in resistance training for healthy adults. Med Sci Sports Exerc. 2002 Feb;34(2):364-80

101 Campos GE, Luecke TJ, Wendeln HK, Toma K, Hagerman FC, Murray TF, Ragg KE, Ratamess NA, Kraemer WJ, Staron RS. Muscular adaptations in response to three different resistance-training regimens: specificity of repetition maximum training zones. Eur J Appl Physiol. 2002 Nov;88(1-2):50-60

102 McCaulley GO, McBride JM, Cormie P, Hudson MB, Nuzzo JL, Quindry JC, Travis Triplett N. Acute hormonal and neuromuscular responses to hypertrophy, strength and power type resistance exercise. Eur J Appl Physiol. 2009 Mar;105(5):695-704

103 Crewther B, Cronin J, Keogh J, Cook C. The salivary testosterone and cortisol response to three loading schemes. J Strength Cond Res. 2008 Jan;22(1):250-5

104 Cannon J, Kay D, Tarpenning KM, Marino FE. Comparative effects of resistance training on peak isometric torque, muscle hypertrophy, voluntary activation and surface EMG between young and elderly women. Clin Physiol Funct Imaging. 2007 Mar;27(2):91-100

105 Ahtiainen JP, Pakarinen A, Alen M, Kraemer WJ, Häkkinen K. Muscle hypertrophy, hormonal adaptations and strength development during strength training in strength-trained and untrained men. Eur J Appl Physiol. 2003 Aug;89(6):555-63

106 Kraemer WJ, Häkkinen K, Newton RU, McCormick M, Nindl BC, Volek JS, Gotshalk LA, Fleck SJ, Campbell WW, Gordon SE, Farrell PA, Evans WJ. Acute hormonal responses to heavy resistance exercise in younger and older men. Eur J Appl Physiol Occup Physiol. 1998 Feb;77(3):206-11

107 Knapik JJ, Rieger W, Palkoska F, Van Camp S, Darakjy S. United States Army physical readiness training: rationale and evaluation of the physical training doctrine. J Strength Cond Res. 2009 Jul;23(4):1353-62

108 Harman EA, Gutekunst DJ, Frykman PN, Nindl BC, Alemany JA, Mello RP, Sharp MA. Effects of two different eight-week training programs on military physical performance. J Strength Cond Res. 2008 Mar;22(2):524-34

109 Wolfe BL, LeMura LM, Cole PJ. Quantitative analysis of single- vs. multiple-set programs in resistance training. J Strength Cond Res. 2004 Feb;18(1):35-47

110 Kemmler WK, Lauber D, Engelke K, Weineck J. Effects of single- vs. multiple-set resistance training on maximum strength and body composition in trained postmenopausal women. J Strength Cond Res. 2004 Nov;18(4):689-94

111 Drinkwater EJ, Lawton TW, Lindsell RP, Pyne DB, Hunt PH, McKenna MJ. Training leading to repetition failure enhances bench press strength gains in elite junior athletes. J Strength Cond Res. 2005 May;19(2):382-8

112 Haskell WL, Lee IM, Pate RR, Powell KE, Blair SN, Franklin BA, Macera CA, Heath GW, Thompson PD, Bauman A. Physical activity and public health: updated recommendation for adults from the American College of Sports Medicine and the American Heart Association. Med Sci Sports Exerc. 2007 Aug;39(8):1423-34

113 Holloszy JO, Coyle EF. Adaptations of skeletal muscle to endurance exercise and their metabolic consequences. J Appl Physiol. 1984 Apr;56(4):831-8

114 Coggan AR, Spina RJ, King DS, Rogers MA, Brown M, Nemeth PM, Holloszy JO. Skeletal muscle adaptations to endurance training in 60- to 70-yr-old men and women. J Appl Physiol. 1992 May;72(5):1780-6

115 Baggish AL, Wang F, Weiner RB, Elinoff JM, Tournoux F, Boland A, Picard MH, Hutter AM Jr, Wood MJ. Training-specific changes in cardiac structure and function: a prospective and longitudinal assessment of competitive athletes. J Appl Physiol. 2008 Apr;104(4):1121-8

116 McArdle WD, Katch FI, Katch VL. Chapter 7, Energy transfer in exercise, in Exercise Physiology: energy, nutrition, and human performance, 5th ed., Baltimore, Maryland: Lippincott Williams & Wilkins, 2001, p. 162

117 Donnelly JE, Blair SN, Jakicic JM, Manore MM, Rankin JW, Smith BK; American College of Sports Medicine. American College of Sports Medicine Position Stand. Appropriate physical activity intervention strategies for weight loss and prevention of weight regain for adults. Med Sci Sports Exerc. 2009 Feb;41(2):459-71

118 Brouns F, van der Vusse GJ. Utilization of lipids during exercise in human subjects: metabolic and dietary constraints. Br J Nutr. 1998 Feb;79(2):117-28

119 Martin WH 3rd. Effects of acute and chronic exercise on fat metabolism. Exerc Sport Sci Rev. 1996;24:203-31

120 Westerterp KR, Meijer GA, Schoffelen P, Janssen EM. Body mass, body composition and sleeping metabolic rate before, during and after endurance training. Eur J Appl Physiol Occup Physiol. 1994;69(3):203-8

121 Kohrt WM, Obert KA, Holloszy JO. Exercise training improves fat distribution patterns in 60- to 70-year-old men and women. J Gerontol. 1992 Jul;47(4):M99-105

122 Carter SL, Rennie CD, Hamilton SJ, Tarnopolsky. Changes in skeletal muscle in males and females following endurance training. Can J Physiol Pharmacol. 2001 May;79(5):386-92

123 Sillanpää E, Häkkinen A, Nyman K, Mattila M, Cheng S, Karavirta L, Laaksonen DE, Huuhka N, Kraemer WJ, Häkkinen K. Body composition and fitness during strength and/or endurance training in older men. Med Sci Sports Exerc. 2008 May;40(5):950-8

124 Paoli A, Pacelli F, Bargossi AM, Marcolin G, Guzzinati S, Neri M, Bianco A, Palma A. Effects of three distinct protocols of fitness training on body composition, strength and blood lactate. J Sports Med Phys Fitness. 2010 Mar;50(1):43-51

125 Sanal E, Ardic F, Kirac S. Effects of aerobic or combined aerobic resistance exercise on body composition in overweight and obese adults: gender differences. a randomized intervention study. Eur J Phys Rehabil Med. 2012 May 8

126 Pierson LM, Herbert WG, Norton HJ, Kiebzak GM, Griffith P, Fedor JM, Ramp WK, Cook JW. Effects of combined aerobic and resistance training versus aerobic training alone in cardiac rehabilitation. J Cardiopulm Rehabil. 2001 Mar-Apr;21(2):101-10

127 Dolezal BA, Potteiger JA. Concurrent resistance and endurance training influence basal metabolic rate in nondieting individuals. J Appl Physiol. 1998 Aug;85(2):695-700

128 Park SK, Park JH, Kwon YC, Kim HS, Yoon MS, Park HT. The effect of combined aerobic and resistance exercise training on abdominal fat in obese middle-aged women. J Physiol Anthropol Appl Human Sci. 2003 May;22(3):129-35

129 Bryner RW, Ullrich IH, Sauers J, Donley D, Hornsby G, Kolar M, Yeater R. Effects of resistance vs. aerobic training combined with an 800 calorie liquid diet on lean body mass and resting metabolic rate. J Am Coll Nutr. 1999 Apr;18(2):115-21

130 Segal KR, Gutin B. Thermic effects of food and exercise in lean and obese women. Metabolism. 1983 Jun;32(6):581-9

131 Stiegler P, Cunliffe A. The role of diet and exercise for the maintenance of fat-free mass and resting metabolic rate during weight loss. Sports Med. 2006;36(3):239-62

132 Schuenke MD, Mikat RP, McBride JM. Effect of an acute period of resistance exercise on excess post-exercise oxygen consumption: implications for body mass management. Eur J Appl Physiol. 2002 Mar;86(5):411-7

133 West DW, Burd NA, Staples AW, Phillips SM. Human exercise-mediated skeletal muscle hypertrophy is an intrinsic process. Int J Biochem Cell Biol. 2010 Sep;42(9):1371-5

134 Fahey TD, Rolph R, Moungmee P, Nagel J, Mortara S. Serum testosterone, body composition, and strength of young adults. Med Sci Sports. 1976 Spring;8(1):31-4

135 Kraemer WJ, Gordon SE, Fleck SJ, Marchitelli LJ, Mello R, Dziados JE, Friedl K, Harman E, Maresh C, Fry AC. Endogenous anabolic hormonal and growth factor responses to heavy resistance exercise in males and females. Int J Sports Med. 1991 Apr;12(2):228-35

136 Wheeler GD, Wall SR, Belcastro AN, Cumming DC. Reduced serum testosterone and prolactin levels in male distance runners. JAMA. 1984 Jul 27;252(4):514-6

137 Hackney AC. Effects of endurance exercise on the reproductive system of men: the "exercise-hypogonadal male condition". J Endocrinol Invest. 2008 Oct;31(10):932-8

138 O'Keefe JH, Patil HR, Lavie CJ, Magalski A, Vogel RA, McCullough PA. Potential adverse cardiovascular effects from excessive endurance exercise. Mayo Clin Proc. 2012 Jun;87(6):587-95

139 Sayers SP, Gibson K, Cook CR. Effect of high-speed power training on muscle performance, function, and pain in older adults with knee osteoarthritis: a pilot investigation. Arthritis Care Res (Hoboken). 2012 Jan;64(1):46-53

[140] Jansson E, Kaijser L. Muscle adaptation to extreme endurance training in man. Acta Physiol Scand. 1977 Jul;100(3):315-24

[141] Thorstensson A, Larsson L, Tesch P, Karlsson J. Muscle strength and fiber composition in athletes and sedentary men. Med Sci Sports. 1977 Spring;9(1):26-30

[142] Kraemer WJ. Endocrine responses and adaptations to resistance exercise. Medicine Science Sports Exercise. Med Sci Sports Exerc. 1988 Oct;20(5 Suppl):S152-7; Kraemer WJ, Marchitelli L, McCurry D, Mello R, Dziados JE, Harman E, Frykman P, Gordon SE, Fleck SJ. Hormonal and growth factor responses to heavy resistance exercise. Journal of Applied Physiology. J Appl Physiol. 1990 Oct;69(4):1442-50

[143] Buresh R, Berg K, French J. The effect of resistive exercise rest interval on hormonal response, strength, and hypertrophy with training. J Strength Cond Res. 2009 Jan;23(1):62-71

[144] Westcott WL, Winett RA, Anderson ES, Wojcik JR, Loud RL, Cleggett E, Glover S. Effects of regular and slow speed resistance training on muscle strength. J Sports Med Phys Fitness. 2001 Jun;41(2):154-8

[145] Tanimoto M, Ishii N. Effects of low-intensity resistance exercise with slow movement and tonic force generation on muscular function in young men. J Appl Physiol. 2006 Apr;100(4):1150-7

[146] Tanimoto M, Kawano H, Gando Y, Sanada K, Yamamoto K, Ishii N, Tabata I, Miyachi M. Low-intensity resistance training with slow movement and tonic force generation increases basal limb blood flow. Clin Physiol Funct Imaging. 2009 Apr;29(2):128-35

[147] Watanabe Y, Tanimoto M, Ohgane A, Sanada K, Miyachi M, Ishii N. Low-intensity Resistance Exercise with Slow Movement and Tonic Force Generation Increases Muscle Size and Strength in Older Adults. J Aging Phys Act. 2012 Jul 24

[148] Seger JY, Thorstensson A. Effects of eccentric versus concentric training on thigh muscle strength and EMG. Int J Sports Med. 2005 Jan-Feb;26(1):45-52

[149] Zaras N, Spengos K, Methenitis S, Papadopoulos C, Karampatsos G, Georgiadis G, Stasinaki A, Manta P, Terzis G. Effects of Strength vs. Ballistic-Power Training on Throwing Performance. J Sports Sci Med. 2013 Mar 1;12(1):130-7

[150] Winchester JB, McBride JM, Maher MA, Mikat RP, Allen BK, Kline DE, McGuigan MR. Eight weeks of ballistic exercise improves power independently of changes in strength and muscle fiber type expression. J Strength Cond Res. 2008 Nov;22(6):1728-3

[151] Nosaka K, Sakamoto K, Newton M, Sacco P. How long does the protective effect on eccentric exercise-induced muscle damage last? Med Sci Sports Exerc. 2001 Sep;33(9):1490-5

[152] Chatzinikolaou A, Fatouros IG, Gourgoulis V, Avloniti A, Jamurtas AZ, Nikolaidis MG, Douroudos I, Michailidis Y, Beneka A, Malliou P, Tofas T, Georgiadis I, Mandalidis D, Taxildaris K. Time course of changes in performance and inflammatory responses after acute plyometric exercise. J Strength Cond Res. 2010 May;24(5):1389-98

[153] Howard RL. Plyometric concepts reinvent lower extremity rehabilitation. Biomechanics, September, 2004, http://www.biomech.com/showArticle.jhtml?articleID=47902582

[154] Turner AM, Owings M, Schwane J. Improvement in running economy after 6 weeks of plyometric training. Journal of Strength and Conditioning Research, 2003, 17(1), 60-67

[155] Masamoto N, Larson R, Gates T, Faigenbaum A. Acute effects of plyometric exercise on maximum squat performance in male athletes. Journal of Strength and conditioning Research, 2003, 17(1), 68-71

[156] Hamilton AJ, Haier RJ, Buchsbaum MS, 1984. Intrinsic enjoyment and boredom coping scales: validation with personality, evoked potential and attention measures. Personality and individual differences 5 (2), 183-193

[157] R Demak. Mysterious malady. Sports Illustrated. 74(13):44-49. 1991

[158] Porter JM, Wu WF, Crossley RM, Knopp SW, Campbell OC. Adopting an external focus of attention improves sprinting performance in low-skilled sprinters. J Strength Cond Res. 2015 Apr;29(4):947-53

[159] Stone MH. Muscle conditioning and muscle injuries. Med Sci Sports Exerc. 1990 Aug;22(4):457-62

160 Yamamoto LM, Lopez RM, Klau JF, Casa DJ, Kraemer WJ, Maresh CM. The effects of resistance training on endurance distance running performance among highly trained runners: a systematic review. J Strength Cond Res. 2008 Nov;22(6):2036-44

161 Kraemer WJ, Adams K, Cafarelli E, Dudley GA, Dooly C, Feigenbaum MS, Fleck SJ, Franklin B, Fry AC, Hoffman JR, Newton RU, Potteiger J, Stone MH, Ratamess NA, Triplett-McBride T; American College of Sports Medicine. American College of Sports Medicine position stand. Progression models in resistance training for healthy adults. Med Sci Sports Exerc. 2002 Feb;34(2):364-80

162 Issurin V. Block periodization versus traditional training theory: a review. J Sports Med Phys Fitness. 2008 Mar;48(1):65-75

163 Monteiro AG, Aoki MS, Evangelista AL, Alveno DA, Monteiro GA, Piçarro Ida C, Ugrinowitsch C. Nonlinear periodization maximizes strength gains in split resistance training routines. J Strength Cond Res. 2009 Jul;23(4):1321-6

164 Luebbers PE, Potteiger JA, Hulver MW, Thyfault JP, Carper MJ, Lockwood RH. Effects of plyometric training and recovery on vertical jump performance and anaerobic strength. J Strength Cond Res. 2003 Nov;17(4):704-9

165 Newton RU, Rogers RA, Volek JS, Häkkinen K, Kraemer WJ. Four weeks of optimal load ballistic resistance training at the end of season attenuates declining jump performance of women volleyball players. J Strength Cond Res. 2006 Nov;20(4):955-61

166 Palmer CD, Sleivert GG. Running economy is impaired following a single bout of resistance exercise. J Sci Med Sport. 2001 Dec;4(4):447-59

167 Sporer BC, Wenger HA. Effects of aerobic exercise on strength performance following various periods of recovery. Journal of Strength and Conditioning Research. 2003 17(4)638-644

168 Davis WJ, Wood DT, Andrews RG, Elkind LM, Davis WB. Concurrent training enhances athletes' strength, muscle endurance, and other measures. J Strength Cond Res. 2008 Sep;22(5):1487-502

169 Leveritt M, Abernethy PJ, Barry BK, Logan PA. Concurrent strength and endurance training. A review. Sports Med. 1999 Dec;28(6):413-27

170 Kraemer WJ, Patton JF, Gordon SE, Harman EA, Deschenes MR, Reynolds K, Newton RU, Triplett NT, Dziados JE. Compatibility of high-intensity strength and endurance training on hormonal and skeletal muscle adaptations. J Appl Physiol. 1995 Mar;78(3):976-89

171 Hather BM, Tesch PA, Buchanan P, Dudley GA. Influence of eccentric actions on skeletal muscle adaptations to resistance training. Acta Physiol. Scand. 1991;143:177-185

172 Staron RS, Leonardi MJ, Karapondo DL, Malicky ES, Falkel JE, Hagerman FC, Hikida RS. Strength and skeletal muscle adaptations in heavy-resistance trained women after detraining and retraining. J. Appl. Physiol. 1991;70:631-640

173 Doherty RA, Neary JP, Bhambhani YN, Wenger HA. Fifteen-day cessation of training on selected physiological and performance variables in women runners. J Strength Cond Res. 2003 Aug;17(3):599-607

174 Donnelly JE, Smith B, Jacobsen DJ, Kirk E, Dubose K, Hyder M, Bailey B, Washburn R. The role of exercise for weight loss and maintenance. Best Pract Res Clin Gastroenterol. 2004 Dec;18(6):1009-29

175 Bloomer RJ. Energy cost of moderate-duration resistance and aerobic exercise. J Strength Cond Res. 2005 Nov;19(4):878-82

176 Avila JJ, Gutierres JA, Sheehy ME, Lofgren IE, Delmonico MJ. Effect of moderate intensity resistance training during weight loss on body composition and physical performance in overweight older adults. Eur J Appl Physiol. 2010 Jun;109(3):517-25

177 Office of the Surgeon General (US); Office of Disease Prevention and Health Promotion (US); Centers for Disease Control and Prevention (US); National Institutes of Health (US). The Surgeon General's Call To Action To Prevent and Decrease Overweight and Obesity. Rockville (MD): Office of the Surgeon General (US); 2001

[178] Grund A, Krause H, Kraus M, Siewers M, Rieckert H, Müller MJ. Association between different attributes of physical activity and fat mass in untrained, endurance- and resistance-trained men. Eur J Appl Physiol. 2001 Apr;84(4):310-20

[179] Hunter GR, McCarthy JP, Bamman MM. Effects of resistance training on older adults. Sports Med. 2004;34(5):329-48

[180] Brunner F, Schmid A, Sheikhzadeh A, Nordin M, Yoon J, Frankel V. Effects of aging on Type II muscle fibers: a systematic review of the literature. J Aging Phys Act. 2007 Jul;15(3):336-48

[181] Aoyagi Y, Shephard RJ. Aging and muscle function. Sports Med. 1992 Dec;14(6):376-96

[182] Buford TW, Rossi SJ, Smith DB, Warren AJ. A comparison of periodization models during nine weeks with equated volume and intensity for strength. J Strength Cond Res. 2007 Nov;21(4):1245-50

[183] Hoffman JR, Wendell M, Cooper J, Kang J. Comparison between linear and nonlinear in-season training programs in freshman football players. Strength Cond Res. 2003 Aug;17(3):561-5

[184] Rhea MR, Phillips WT, Burkett LN, Stone WJ, Ball SD, Alvar BA, Thomas AB. A comparison of linear and daily undulating periodized programs with equated endurance and intensity for local muscle endurance. Journal of Strength and Conditioning Research, 2003, 17(1):82-87

[185] Paluska SA, Schwenk TL. Physical activity and mental health: current concepts. Sports Med. 2000 Mar;29(3):167-80

[186] McKenzie DC. Markers of excessive exercise. Can J Appl Physiol. 1999 Feb;24(1):66-73

[187] Nieman DC. Exercise, upper respiratory tract infection, and the immune system. Med Sci Sports Exerc. 1994 Feb;26(2):128-39

[188] Moreira A, Delgado L, Moreira P, Haahtela T. Does exercise increase the risk of upper respiratory tract infections? Br Med Bull. 2009;90:111-31

[189] Weidner TG, Cranston T, Schurr T, Kaminsky LA. The effect of exercise training on the severity and duration of a viral upper respiratory illness. Med Sci Sports Exerc. 1998 Nov;30(11):1578-83

[190] Weidner T, Schurr T. Effect of exercise on upper respiratory tract infection in sedentary subjects. Br J Sports Med. 2003 Aug;37(4):304-6

[191] Ackerman J. Ah-choo! The uncommon life of the common cold. Twelve, Hachette Book Group. New York, 2010. p. 162

[192] Izquierdo M, Ibañez J, González-Badillo JJ, Ratamess NA, Kraemer WJ, Häkkinen K, Bonnabau H, Granados C, French DN, Gorostiaga EM. Detraining and tapering effects on hormonal responses and strength performance. J Strength Cond Res. 2007 Aug;21(3):768-75

[193] Fradkin AJ, Zazryn TR, Smoliga JM. Effects of warming-up on physical performance: a systematic review with meta-analysis. J Strength Cond Res. 2010 Jan;24(1):140-8

[194] Canadian Standardized Test of Fitness (CSTF) Operations Manual, 3rd ed., as reprinted in ACSM's Guidelines for Exercise Testing and Prescription, 6th ed., by the American College of Sports Medicine, 2000, p 85

[195] Baechle, TR, National Strength and Conditioning Association. Essentials of Strength and Conditioning. Champaign, IL: Human Kinetics, 1994, p. 427

[196] Paulsen G, Myklestad D, Raastad T. The influence of volume of exercise on early adaptations to strength training. J Strength Cond Res. 2003 Feb;17(1):115-20

[197] Rønnestad BR, Egeland W, Kvamme NH, Refsnes PE, Kadi F, Raastad T. Dissimilar effects of one- and three-set strength training on strength and muscle mass gains in upper and lower body in untrained subjects. J Strength Cond Res. 2007 Feb;21(1):157-63

[198] Mangine GT, Ratamess NA, Hoffman JR, Faigenbaum AD, Kang J, Chilakos A. The effects of combined ballistic and heavy resistance training on maximal lower- and upper-body strength in recreationally trained men. J Strength Cond Res. 2008 Jan;22(1):132-9

199 Robbins DW, Marshall PW, McEwen M. The effect of training volume on lower-body strength. J Strength Cond Res. 2012 Jan;26(1):34-9

200 Rubenstein LZ, Josephson KR. Interventions to reduce the multifactorial risks for falling. In: Masdeu JC, Sudarsky L. Gait Disorders and Aging: falls and therapeutic strategies. Philadelphia: Lippincott-Raven, 1997, pp. 300-326

201 Cheung K, Hume P, Maxwell L. Delayed onset muscle soreness : treatment strategies and performance factors. Sports Med. 2003;33(2):145-64

202 Fogelholm M, Kukkonen-Harjula K, Nenonen A, Pasanen M. Effects of walking training on weight maintenance after a very-low-energy diet in premenopausal obese women: a randomized controlled trial. Arch Intern Med. 2000 Jul 24;160(14):2177-84

203 Moreau KL, Degarmo R, Langley J, McMahon C, Howley ET, Bassett DR Jr, Thompson DL. Increasing daily walking lowers blood pressure in postmenopausal women. Med Sci Sports Exerc. 2001 Nov;33(11):1825-31

204 Kai MC, Anderson M, Lau EM. Exercise interventions: defusing the world's osteoporosis time bomb. Bull World Health Organ. 2003;81(11):827-30

205 Tanne JH. Walking protects elderly people from dementia, studies show. BMJ. 2004 Oct 2;329(7469):761. http://bmj.bmjjournals.com/cgi/content/full/329/7469/761-c

206 Heggie J. Running with the whole body: a 30-day program to running faster with less effort. Berkeley, California: Somatic Resources and North Atlantic Books, 1996

207 Ekkekakis P, Hall EE, Petruzzello SJ. Practical markers of the transition from aerobic to anaerobic metabolism during exercise: rationale and a case for affect-based exercise prescription. Prev Med. 2004 Feb;38(2):149-59

208 Williams PT. Relationship of distance run per week to coronary heart disease risk factors in 8,283 male runners: the National Runners' Health Study. Archives of Internal Medicine. 157(2):191-198

209 Bishop D, Girard O, Mendez-Villanueva A. Repeated-sprint ability - part II: recommendations for training. Sports Med. 2011 Sep 1;41(9):741-56

210 Sevits KJ, Melanson EL, Swibas T, Binns SE, Klochak AL, Lonac MC, Peltonen GL, Scalzo RL, Schweder MM, Smith AM, Wood LM, Melby CL, Bell C. Total daily energy expenditure is increased following a single bout of sprint interval training. Physiol Rep. 2013 Oct;1(5):e00131

211 Muir J. Our national parks. Boston: Houghton Mifflin and Company, 1901. http://www.sierraclub.org/john_muir_exhibit

212 Greie S, Humpeler E, Gunga HC, Koralewski E, Klingler A, Mittermayr M, Fries D, Lechleitner M, Hoertnagl H, Hoffmann G, Strauss-Blasche G, Schobersberger W. Improvement of metabolic syndrome markers through altitude specific hiking vacations. J Endocrinol Invest. 2006 Jun;29(6):497-504

213 The Mother Nature Network. 5 Reasons Not to Drink Bottled Water: it's expensive, wasteful, and — contrary to popular belief — not any healthier for you than tap water. http://www.mnn.com/food/healthy-eating/stories/5-reasons-not-to-drink-bottled-water

214 Hu Z, Morton LW, Mahler RL. Bottled water: United States consumers and their perceptions of water quality. Int J Environ Res Public Health. 2011 Feb;8(2):565-78

215 Boschmann M, Steiniger J, Franke G, Birkenfeld AL, Luft FC, Jordan J. Water drinking induces thermogenesis through osmosensitive mechanisms. J Clin Endocrinol Metab. 2007 Aug;92(8):3334-7

216 Benton D. Dehydration influences mood and cognition: a plausible hypothesis? Nutrients. 2011 May;3(5):555-73

217 Valtin H. "Drink at least eight glasses of water a day." Really? Is there scientific evidence for "8 x 8"? Am J Physiol Regul Integr Comp Physiol. 2002 Nov;283(5):R993-1004

218 Sawka MN, Cheuvront SN, Carter R 3rd. Human water needs. Nutr Rev. 2005 Jun;63(6 Pt 2):S30-9

219 Almond CS, Shin AY, Fortescue EB, Mannix RC, Wypij D, Binstadt BA, Duncan CN, Olson DP, Salerno AE, Newburger JW, Greenes DS. Hyponatremia among runners in the Boston Marathon. N Engl J Med. 2005 Apr

14;352(15):1550-6

[220] Ballantyne, C. Strange but true: drinking too much water can kill, in Scientific American, June 21, 2007. http://www.scientificamerican.com/article.cfm?id=strange-but-true-drinking-too-much-water-can-kill

[221] Bilsborough SA, Crowe TC. Low-carbohydrate diets: what are the potential short- and long-term health implications? Asia Pac J Clin Nutr. 2003;12(4):396-404

[222] Willett WC, The Harvard School of Public Health. Eat, Drink, and Be Healthy. New York: Simon & Schuster, 2001, p. 95

[223] Salmeron J, Ascherio A, Rimm EB, Colditz GA, Spiegelman D, Jenkins DJ, Stampfer MJ, Wing AL, Willett WC. Dietary fiber, glycemic load, and risk of NIDDM in men. Diabetes Care. 1997 Apr;20(4):545-50

[224] Salmeron J, Manson JE, Stampfer MJ, Colditz GA, Wing AL, Willett WC. Dietary fiber, glycemic load, and risk of non-insulin-dependent diabetes mellitus in women. JAMA. 1997 Feb 12;277(6):472-7

[225] Murakami K, Okubo H, Sasaki S. Effect of dietary factors on incidence of type 2 diabetes: a systematic review of cohort studies. J Nutr Sci Vitaminol (Tokyo). 2005 Aug;51(4):292-310

[226] The Oregon State University Linus Pauling Institute Micronutrient Information Center. Glycemic index and glycemic load. http://lpi.oregonstate.edu/infocenter/foods/grains/gigl.html

[227] Nettleton JA, Steffen LM, Ni H, Liu K, Jacobs DR Jr. Dietary patterns and risk of incident type 2 diabetes in the Multi-Ethnic Study of Atherosclerosis (MESA). Diabetes Care. 2008 Sep;31(9):1777-82

[228] McArdle WD, Katch FI, Katch VL. Exercise physiology: energy, nutrition, and human performance, 5th ed., Baltimore, Maryland: Lippincott Williams & Wilkins, 2001, page 840

[229] Bray GA, Popkin BM. Dietary fat intake does affect obesity! Am J Clin Nutr. 1998 Dec;68(6):1157-73

[230] Astrup A. The role of dietary fat in obesity. Semin Vasc Med. 2005 Feb;5(1):40-7

[231] Sacks FM, Bray GA, Carey VJ, Smith SR, Ryan DH, Anton SD, McManus K, Champagne CM, Bishop LM, Laranjo N, Leboff MS, Rood JC, de Jonge L, Greenway FL, Loria CM, Obarzanek E, Williamson DA. Comparison of weight-loss diets with different compositions of fat, protein, and carbohydrates. N Engl J Med. 2009 Feb 26;360(9):859-73

[232] Willett WC, Leibel RL. Dietary fat is not a major determinant of body fat. Am J Med. 2002 Dec 30;113 Suppl 9B:47S-59S

[233] McArdle WD, Katch FI, Katch VL. Chapter 3, Optimal nutrition for exercise, in Exercise physiology: energy, nutrition, and human performance, 5th ed., Baltimore, Maryland: Lippincott Williams & Wilkins, 2001, page 83

[234] Fraser GE, Bennett HW, Jaceldo KB, Sabate J. Effect on body weight of a free 76 Kilojoule (320 calorie) daily supplement of almonds for six months. J Am Coll Nutr. 2002 Jun;21(3):275-83

[235] Johnson ML, Burke BS, Mayer J. Relative importance of inactivity and overeating in the energy balance of obese high school girls. Am J Clin Nutr. 1956 Jan-Feb;4(1):37-44

[236] Esmarck B, Andersen JL, Olsen S, Richter EA, Mizuno M, Kjaer M. Timing of postexercise protein intake is important for muscle hypertrophy with resistance training in elderly humans. J Physiol. 2001 Aug 15;535(Pt 1):301-11

[237] Johnstone AM, Shannon E, Whybrow S, Reid CA, Stubbs RJ. Altering the temporal distribution of energy intake with isoenergetically dense foods given as snacks does not affect total daily energy intake in normal-weight men. Br J Nutr. 2000 Jan;83(1):7-14

[238] Leidy HJ, Campbell WW. The effect of eating frequency on appetite control and food intake: brief synopsis of controlled feeding studies. J Nutr. 2011 Jan;141(1):154-7

[239] Patel SR. Reduced sleep as an obesity risk factor. Obes Rev. 2009 Nov;10 Suppl 2:61-8

[240] Farshchi HR, Taylor MA, Macdonald IA. Decreased thermic effect of food after an irregular compared with a regular meal pattern in healthy lean women. Int J Obes Relat Metab Disord. 2004 May;28(5):653-60

[241] Hall WL. Dietary saturated and unsaturated fats as determinants of blood pressure and vascular function. Nutr

Res Rev. 2009 Jun;22(1):18-38

242 McGill HC Jr, McMahan CA, Zieske AW, Tracy RE, Malcom GT, Herderick EE, Strong JP. Association of Coronary Heart Disease Risk Factors with microscopic qualities of coronary atherosclerosis in youth. Circulation. 2000 Jul 25;102(4):374-9

243 Lopez-Garcia E, Schulze MB, Meigs JB, Manson JE, Rifai N, Stampfer MJ, Willett WC, Hu FB. Consumption of trans fatty acids is related to plasma biomarkers of inflammation and endothelial dysfunction. J Nutr. 2005 Mar;135(3):562-6

244 Grenon SM, Conte MS, Nosova E, Alley H, Chong K, Harris WS, Vittinghoff E, Owens CD. Association between n-3 polyunsaturated fatty acid content of red blood cells and inflammatory biomarkers in patients with peripheral artery disease. J Vasc Surg. 2013 Nov;58(5):1283-90

245 Schwalfenberg G. Omega-3 fatty acids: their beneficial role in cardiovascular health. Can Fam Physician. 2006 Jun;52:734-40

246 Simopoulos AP. Omega-3 fatty acids in inflammation and autoimmune diseases. J Am Coll Nutr. 2002 Dec;21(6):495-505

247 Sanjoaquin MA, Appleby PN, Thorogood M, Mann JI, Key TJ. Nutrition, lifestyle and colorectal cancer incidence: a prospective investigation of 10998 vegetarians and non-vegetarians in the United Kingdom. Br J Cancer. 2004 Jan 12;90(1):118-21

248 Cohen JH, Kristal AR, Stanford JL. Fruit and vegetable intakes and prostate cancer risk. J Natl Cancer Inst. 2000 Jan 5;92(1):61-8

249 Perry NS, Houghton PJ, Sampson J, Theobald AE, Hart S, Lis-Balchin M, Hoult JR, Evans P, Jenner P, Milligan S, Perry EK. In-vitro activity of S. lavandulaefolia (Spanish sage) relevant to treatment of Alzheimer's disease. J Pharm Pharmacol. 2001 Oct;53(10):1347-56

250 Tsai CJ, Leitzmann MF, Willett WC, Giovannucci EL. Dietary protein and the risk of cholecystectomy in a cohort of US women: the Nurses' Health Study. Am J Epidemiol. 2004 Jul 1;160(1):11-8

251 Cho E, Seddon JM, Rosner B, Willett WC, Hankinson SE. Prospective study of intake of fruits, vegetables, vitamins, and carotenoids and risk of age-related maculopathy. Arch Ophthalmol. 2004 Jun;122(6):883-92

252 Giovannucci E. Tomatoes, tomato-based products, lycopene, and cancer: review of the epidemiologic literature. J Natl Cancer Inst. 1999 Feb 17;91(4):317-31

253 Hwang ES, Bowen PE. Can the consumption of tomatoes or lycopene reduce cancer risk? Integr Cancer Ther. 2002 Jun;1(2):121-32

254 Basu A, Imrhan V. Tomatoes versus lycopene in oxidative stress and carcinogenesis: conclusions from clinical trials. Eur J Clin Nutr. 2007 Mar;61(3):295-303

255 Weisburger JH. Lycopene and tomato products in health promotion. Exp Biol Med (Maywood). 2002 Nov;227(10):924-7

256 Panel on Macronutrients, Subcommittees on Upper Reference Levels of Nutrients and Interpretation and Uses of Dietary Reference Intakes, and the Standing Committee on the Scientific Evaluation of Dietary Reference Intakes. Dietary Reference Intakes for Energy, Carbohydrate, Fiber, Fat, Fatty Acids, Cholesterol, Protein, and Amino Acids (Macronutrients). The National Academies Press, 2002. http://www.nap.edu/catalog/10490.html

257 Rand WM, Pellett PL, Young VR. Meta-analysis of nitrogen balance studies for estimating protein requirements in healthy adults. Am J Clin Nutr. 2003 Jan;77(1):109-27

258 National Center for Health Statistics, Centers for Disease Control and Prevention, U.S. Department of Health and Human Services. National Health and Nutrition Examination Survey (NHANES): 1999-2004. http://www.cdc.gov/nchs/data/nhanes/databriefs/calories.pdf

259 Cermak NM, Res PT, de Groot LC, Saris WH, van Loon LJ. Protein supplementation augments the adaptive response of skeletal muscle to resistance-type exercise training: a meta-analysis. Am J Clin Nutr. 2012 Dec;96(6):1454-64

260 Tieland M, Dirks ML, van der Zwaluw N, Verdijk LB, van de Rest O, de Groot LC, van Loon LJ. Protein supplementation increases muscle mass gain during prolonged resistance-type exercise training in frail elderly people: a randomized, double-blind, placebo-controlled trial. J Am Med Dir Assoc. 2012 Oct;13(8):713-9

261 Thompson BJ, Ryan ED, Sobolewski EJ, Smith-Ryan AE. Dietary protein intake is associated with maximal and explosive strength of the leg flexors in young and older blue collar workers. Nutr Res. 2015 Apr;35(4):280-6

262 Tang JE, Phillips SM. Maximizing muscle protein anabolism: the role of protein quality. Curr Opin Clin Nutr Metab Care. 2009 Jan;12(1):66-71

263 Weigle DS, Breen PA, Matthys CC, Callahan HS, Meeuws KE, Burden VR, Purnell JQ. A high-protein diet induces sustained reductions in appetite, ad libitum caloric intake, and body weight despite compensatory changes in diurnal plasma leptin and ghrelin concentrations. Am J Clin Nutr. 2005 Jul;82(1):41-8

264 Reuters Health News. "High-protein diets curb appetite." http://au.health.yahoo.com/050722/3/66u6.html?r=967438252

265 Nelson LH, Tucker LA. Diet composition related to body fat in a multivariate study of 203 men. J Am Diet Assoc. 1996 Aug;96(8):771-7

266 Astrup A, Meinert Larsen T, Harper A. Atkins and other low-carbohydrate diets: hoax or an effective tool for weight loss? Lancet. 2004 Sep 4;364(9437):897-9

267 Feskanich D, Willett WC, Stampfer MJ, Colditz GA. Protein consumption and bone fractures in women. Am J Epidemiol. 1996 Mar 1;143(5):472-9

268 Allen LH, Bartlett RS, Block GD. Reduction of renal calcium reabsorption in man by consumption of dietary protein. J Nutr. 1979 Aug;109(8):1345-50

269 Schwingshackl L, Hoffmann G. Comparison of high vs. normal/low protein diets on renal function in subjects without chronic kidney disease: a systematic review and meta-analysis. PLoS One. 2014 May 22;9(5):e97656

270 Marckmann P, Osther P, Pedersen AN, Jespersen B. High-protein diets and renal health. J Ren Nutr. 2015 Jan;25(1):1-5

271 Hariharan D, Vellanki K, Kramer H. The Western diet and chronic kidney disease. Curr Hypertens Rep. 2015 Apr;17(4):529

272 Giannini S, Nobile M, Sartori L, Dalle Carbonare L, Ciuffreda M, Corro P, D'Angelo A, Calo L, Crepaldi G. Acute effects of moderate dietary protein restriction in patients with idiopathic hypercalciuria and calcium nephrolithiasis. Am J Clin Nutr. 1999 Feb;69(2):267-71

273 Rotily M, Leonetti F, Iovanna C, Berthezene P, Dupuy P, Vazi A, Berland Y. Effects of low animal protein or high-fiber diets on urine composition in calcium nephrolithiasis. Kidney Int. 2000 Mar;57(3):1115-23

274 Borghi L, Schianchi T, Meschi T, Guerra A, Allegri F, Maggiore U, Novarini A. Comparison of two diets for the prevention of recurrent stones in idiopathic hypercalciuria. N Engl J Med. 2002 Jan 10;346(2):77-84

275 Tracy CR, Best S, Bagrodia A, Poindexter JR, Adams-Huet B, Sakhaee K, Maalouf N, Pak CY, Pearle MS. Animal protein and the risk of kidney stones: a comparative metabolic study of animal protein sources. J Urol. 2014 Jul;192(1):137-41

276 Van Nielen M, Feskens EJ, Mensink M, Sluijs I, Molina E, Amiano P, Ardanaz E, Balkau B, Beulens JW, Boeing H, Clavel-Chapelon F, Fagherazzi G, Franks PW, Halkjaer J, Huerta JM, Katzke V, Key TJ, Khaw KT, Krogh V, Kühn T, Menéndez VV, Nilsson P, Overvad K, Palli D, Panico S, Rolandsson O, Romieu I, Sacerdote C, Sánchez MJ, Schulze MB, Spijkerman AM, Tjonneland A, Tumino R, van der A DL, Würtz AM, Zamora-Ros R, Langenberg C, Sharp SJ, Forouhi NG, Riboli E, Wareham NJ; InterAct Consortium. Dietary protein intake and

incidence of type 2 diabetes in Europe: the EPIC-InterAct Case-Cohort Study. Diabetes Care. 2014 Jul;37(7):1854-62

[277] Hernández-Alonso P, Salas-Salvadó J, Ruiz-Canela M, Corella D, Estruch R, Fitó M, Arós F, Gómez-Gracia E, Fiol M, Lapetra J, Basora J, Serra-Majem L, Muñoz MÁ, Buil-Cosiales P, Saiz C, Bulló M. High dietary protein intake is associated with an increased body weight and total death risk. Clin Nutr. 2015 Apr 7

[278] Elliott P, Stamler J, Dyer AR, Appel L, Dennis B, Kesteloot H, Ueshima H, Okayama A, Chan Q, Garside DB, Zhou B. Association between protein intake and blood pressure: the INTERMAP Study. Arch Intern Med. 2006 Jan 9;166(1):79-87

[279] Bradbury KE, Crowe FL, Appleby PN, Schmidt JA, Travis RC, Key TJ. Serum concentrations of cholesterol, apolipoprotein A-I and apolipoprotein B in a total of 1694 meat-eaters, fish-eaters, vegetarians and vegans. Eur J Clin Nutr. 2014 Feb;68(2):178-83

[280] Grant R, Bilgin A, Zeuschner C, Guy T, Pearce R, Hokin B, Ashton J. The relative impact of a vegetable-rich diet on key markers of health in a cohort of Australian adolescents. Asia Pac J Clin Nutr. 2008;17(1):107-15

[281] Turner-McGrievy G, Harris M. Key elements of plant-based diets associated with reduced risk of metabolic syndrome. Curr Diab Rep. 2014;14(9):524

[282] Clinton CM, O'Brien S, Law J, Renier CM, Wendt MR. Whole-foods, plant-based diet alleviates the symptoms of osteoarthritis. Arthritis. 2015;2015:708152

[283] Le LT, Sabaté J. Beyond meatless, the health effects of vegan diets: findings from the Adventist cohorts. Nutrients. 2014 May 27;6(6):2131-47

[284] Adlercreutz H. Phytoestrogens: epidemiology and a possible role in cancer protection. Environ Health Perspect. 1995 Oct;103 Suppl 7:103-12

[285] Torabian S, Haddad E, Rajaram S, Banta J, Sabaté J. Acute effect of nut consumption on plasma total polyphenols, antioxidant capacity and lipid peroxidation. J Hum Nutr Diet. 2009 Feb;22(1):64-71

[286] Jones PJ, Raeini-Sarjaz M, Jenkins DJ, Kendall CW, Vidgen E, Trautwein EA, Lapsley KG, Marchie A, Cunnane SC, Connelly PW. Effects of a diet high in plant sterols, vegetable proteins, and viscous fibers (dietary portfolio) on circulating sterol levels and red cell fragility in hypercholesterolemic subjects. Lipids. 2005 Feb;40(2):169-74

[287] Ortega R. Importance of functional foods in the Mediterranean diet. Public Health Nutr. 2006 Dec;9(8A):1136-40

[288] Beer WH, Murray E, Oh SH, Pedersen HE, Wolfe RR, Young VR. A long-term metabolic study to assess the nutritional value of and immunological tolerance to two soy-protein concentrates in adult humans. Am J Clin Nutr. 1989 Nov;50(5):997-1007

[289] U.S. Food and Drug Administration, Code of Federal Regulation, 21CFR101.82, http://www.cfsan.fda.gov/~lrd/cf101-82.html

[290] Arjmandi BH, Khalil DA, Lucas EA, Smith BJ, Sinichi N, Hodges SB, Juma S, Munson ME, Payton ME, Tivis RD, Svanborg A. Soy protein may alleviate osteoarthritis symptoms. Phytomedicine. 2004 Nov;11(7-8):567-75

[291] Zhan S, Ho SC. Meta-analysis of the effects of soy protein containing isoflavones on the lipid profile. Am J Clin Nutr. 2005 Feb;81(2):397-408

[292] Messina MJ. Emerging evidence on the role of soy in reducing prostate cancer risk. Nutr Rev. 2003 Apr;61(4):117-31

[293] McMichael-Phillips DF, Harding C, Morton M, Roberts SA, Howell A, Potten CS, Bundred NJ. Effects of soy-protein supplementation on epithelial proliferation in the histologically normal human breast. Am J Clin Nutr. 1998 Dec;68(6 Suppl):1431S-1435S

[294] Boyapati SM, Shu XO, Ruan ZX, Dai Q, Cai Q, Gao YT, Zheng W. Soyfood intake and breast cancer survival: a followup of the Shanghai Breast Cancer Study. Breast Cancer Res Treat. 2005 Jul;92(1):11-7

[295] Millward DJ. The nutritional value of plant-based diets in relation to human amino acid and protein requirements. Proc Nutr Soc. 1999 May;58(2):249-60

296 Young VR, Pellett PL. Plant proteins in relation to human protein and amino acid nutrition. Am J Clin Nutr. 1994 May;59(5 Suppl):1203S-1212S

297 Butler LM, Sinha R, Millikan RC, Martin CF, Newman B, Gammon MD, Ammerman AS, Sandler RS. Heterocyclic amines, meat intake, and association with colon cancer in a population-based study. Am J Epidemiol. 2003 Mar 1;157(5):434-45

298 Chiu BC, Cerhan JR, Folsom AR, Sellers TA, Kushi LH, Wallace RB, Zheng W, Potter JD. Diet and risk of non-Hodgkin lymphoma in older women. JAMA. 1996 May 1;275(17):1315-21

299 Nicholls SJ, Lundman P, Harmer JA, Cutri B, Griffiths KA, Rye KA, Barter PJ, Celermajer DS. Consumption of saturated fat impairs the anti-inflammatory properties of high-density lipoproteins and endothelial function. J Am Coll Cardiol. 2006 Aug 15;48(4):715-20

300 Stamler J. Diet and coronary heart disease. Biometrics. 1982 Mar;38 Suppl:95-118

301 Berthiaume R, Mandell I, Faucitano L, Lafrenière C. Comparison of alternative beef production systems based on forage finishing or grain-forage diets with or without growth promotants: 1. Feedlot performance, carcass quality, and production costs. J Anim Sci. 2006 Aug;84(8):2168-77

302 Leheska JM, Thompson LD, Howe JC, Hentges E, Boyce J, Brooks JC, Shriver B, Hoover L, Miller MF. Effects of conventional and grass-feeding systems on the nutrient composition of beef. J Anim Sci. 2008 Dec;86(12):3575-85

303 Daley CA, Abbott A, Doyle PS, Nader GA, Larson S. A review of fatty acid profiles and antioxidant content in grass-fed and grain-fed beef. Nutr J. 2010 Mar 10;9:10

304 Spencer EA, Appleby PN, Davey GK, Key TJ. Diet and body mass index in 38000 EPIC-Oxford meat-eaters, fish-eaters, vegetarians and vegans. Int J Obes Relat Metab Disord. 2003 Jun;27(6):728-34

305 Gregory NG. Animal welfare at markets and during transport and slaughter. Meat Sci. 2008 Sep;80(1):2-11

306 Terlouw EM, Arnould C, Auperin B, Berri C, Le Bihan-Duval E, Deiss V, Lefèvre F, Lensink BJ, Mounier L. Pre-slaughter conditions, animal stress and welfare: current status and possible future research. Animal. 2008 Oct;2(10):1501-17

307 Novakofski J, Brewer MS, Mateus-Pinilla N, Killefer J, McCusker RH. Prion biology relevant to bovine spongiform encephalopathy. J Anim Sci. 2005 Jun;83(6):1455-76

308 Swagerty DL Jr, Walling AD, Klein RM. Lactose intolerance. Am Fam Physician. 2002 May 1;65(9):1845-50

309 Demir AU, Karakaya G, Bozkurt B, Sekerel BE, Kalyoncu AF. Asthma and allergic diseases in schoolchildren: third cross-sectional survey in the same primary school in Ankara, Turkey. Pediatr Allergy Immunol. 2004 Dec;15(6):531-8

310 Oranje AP, Wolkerstorfer A, de Waard-van der Spek FB. Natural course of cow's milk allergy in childhood atopic eczema/dermatitis syndrome. Ann Allergy Asthma Immunol. 2002 Dec;89(6 Suppl 1):52-5

311 Arjmandi BH, Khalil DA, Lucas EA, Smith BJ, Sinichi N, Hodges SB, Juma S, Munson ME, Payton ME, Tivis RD, Svanborg A. Soy protein may alleviate osteoarthritis symptoms. Phytomedicine. 2004 Nov;11(7-8):567-75

312 Orimo H. [Calcium intake and osteoporosis]. Clin Calcium. 2004 Nov;14(11):108-10

313 Michaëlsson K, Melhus H, Bellocco R, Wolk A. Dietary calcium and vitamin D intake in relation to osteoporotic fracture risk. Bone. 2003 Jun;32(6):694-703

314 Willett WC, The Harvard School of Public Health. Eat, Drink, and Be Healthy. New York: Simon & Schuster, 2001, p. 143

315 Willett WC, The Harvard School of Public Health. Eat, Drink, and Be Healthy. New York: Simon & Schuster, 2001, p. 142

316 Calbet JA, Dorado C, Diaz-Herrera P, Rodriguez-Rodriguez LP. High femoral bone mineral content and density in male football (soccer) players. Med Sci Sports Exerc. 2001 Oct;33(10):1682-7

317 Mussolino ME, Looker AC, Orwoll ES. Jogging and bone mineral density in men: results from NHANES III. Am J

Public Health. 2001 Jul;91(7):1056-9

[318] Brahm H, Mallmin H, Michaelsson K, Strom H, Ljunghall S. Relationships between bone mass measurements and lifetime physical activity in a Swedish population. Calcif Tissue Int. 1998 May;62(5):400-12

[319] Tseng M, Breslow RA, Graubard BI, Ziegler RG. Dairy, calcium, and vitamin D intakes and prostate cancer risk in the National Health and Nutrition Examination Epidemiologic Follow-up Study cohort. Am J Clin Nutr. 2005 May;81(5):1147-54

[320] Gao X, LaValley MP, Tucker KL. Prospective studies of dairy product and calcium intakes and prostate cancer risk: a meta-analysis. J Natl Cancer Inst. 2005 Dec 7;97(23):1768-77

[321] Aune D, Navarro Rosenblatt DA, Chan DS, Vieira AR, Vieira R, Greenwood DC, Vatten LJ, Norat T. Dairy products, calcium, and prostate cancer risk: a systematic review and meta-analysis of cohort studies. Am J Clin Nutr. 2015 Jan;101(1):87-117

[322] Fairfield KM, Hunter DJ, Colditz GA, Fuchs CS, Cramer DW, Speizer FE, Willett WC, Hankinson SE. A prospective study of dietary lactose and ovarian cancer. Int J Cancer. 2004 Jun 10;110(2):271-7

[323] Lanou AJ. Should dairy be recommended as part of a healthy vegetarian diet? Counterpoint. Am J Clin Nutr. 2009 May;89(5):1638S-1642S

[324] Dudka S, Miller WP. Accumulation of potentially toxic elements in plants and their transfer to human food chain. J Environ Sci Health B. 1999 Jul;34(4):681-708

[325] Tongesayi T, Fedick P, Lechner L, Brock C, Le Beau A, Bray C. Daily bioaccessible levels of selected essential but toxic heavy metals from the consumption of non-dietary food sources. Food Chem Toxicol. 2013 Dec;62:142-7

[326] Ma WC, Denneman W, Faber J. Hazardous exposure of ground-living small mammals to cadmium and lead in contaminated terrestrial ecosystems. Arch Environ Contam Toxicol. 1991 Feb;20(2):266-70

[327] Veltman K, Huijbregts MA, Hamers T, Wijnhoven S, Hendriks AJ. Cadmium accumulation in herbivorous and carnivorous small mammals: meta-analysis of field data and validation of the bioaccumulation model Optimal Modeling for Ecotoxicological Applications. Environ Toxicol Chem. 2007 Jul;26(7):1488-96

[328] Talmage SS, Walton BT. Small mammals as monitors of environmental contaminants. Rev Environ Contam Toxicol. 1991;119:47-145

[329] Mauseth JD, University of Texas, Austin and Universidad Católica, Santiago, Chile. Botany: an introduction to plant biology. Saunders College Publishing, 1991, p. 770

[330] Fontana L, Shew JL, Holloszy JO, Villareal DT. Low bone mass in subjects on a long-term raw vegetarian diet. Arch Intern Med. 2005 Mar 28;165(6):684-9

[331] Messina V, Mangels AR. Considerations in planning vegan diets: children. J Am Diet Assoc. 2001 Jun;101(6):661-9

[332] Barnard ND, Scialli AR, Turner-McGrievy G, Lanou AJ, Glass J. The effects of a low-fat, plant-based dietary intervention on body weight, metabolism, and insulin sensitivity. Am J Med. 2005 Sep;118(9):991-7

[333] Ferrando AA, Green NR. The effect of boron supplementation on lean body mass, plasma testosterone levels, and strength in male bodybuilders. Int J Sport Nutr. 1993 Jun;3(2):140-9

[334] Green NR, Ferrando AA. Plasma boron and the effects of boron supplementation in males. Environ Health Perspect. 1994 Nov;102 Suppl 7:73-7

[335] Vincent JB. Chromium: is it essential, pharmacologically relevant, or toxic? Met Ions Life Sci. 2013;13:171-98

[336] Brown GA, Vukovich MD, Sharp RL, Reifenrath TA, Parsons KA, Effect of oral DHEA on serum testosterone and adaptations to resistance training in young men. J Appl Physiol (1985). 1999 Dec;87(6):2274-83

[337] Muller M, van den Beld AW, van der Schouw YT, Grobbee DE, Lamberts SW. Effects of dehydroepiandrosterone and atamestane supplementation on frailty in elderly men. J Clin Endocrinol Metab. 2006 Oct;91(10):3988-91

[338] Ostojic SM, Calleja J, Jourkesh M. Effects of short-term dehydroepiandrosterone supplementation on body composition in young athletes. Chin J Physiol. 2010 Feb 28;53(1):19-25

[339] Al Balushi RM, Cohen J, Banks M, Paratz JD. The clinical role of glutamine supplementation in patients with multiple trauma: a narrative review. Anaesth Intensive Care. 2013 Jan;41(1):24-34

[340] Wernerman J. Glutamine--from conditionally essential to totally dispensable? Crit Care. 2014 Jul 2;18(4):162

[341] Smedberg M, Wernerman J. Is the glutamine story over? Crit Care. 2016 Nov 10;20(1):361

[342] Waller DP, Martin AM, Farnsworth NR, Awang DV. Lack of androgenicity of Siberian ginseng. JAMA. 1992 May 6;267(17):2329

[343] Secure Nutrition Shop website, http://healthandfitness.com/shop/sns/

[344] Awang DV. Maternal use of ginseng and neonatal androgenization. JAMA. 1991 Jul 17;266(3):363

[345] Ames BN. Low micronutrient intake may accelerate the degenerative diseases of aging through allocation of scarce micronutrients by triage. Proc Natl Acad Sci U S A. 2006 Nov 21;103(47):17589-94

[346] Sanders TA. The nutritional adequacy of plant-based diets. Proc Nutr Soc. 1999 May;58(2):265-9

[347] Craig WJ. Health effects of vegan diets. Am J Clin Nutr. 2009 May;89(5):1627S-1633S

[348] Mądry E, Lisowska A, Grebowiec P, Walkowiak J. The impact of vegan diet on B-12 status in healthy omnivores: five-year prospective study. Acta Sci Pol Technol Aliment. 2012 Apr 2;11(2):209-12

[349] Herrmann W, Geisel J. Vegetarian lifestyle and monitoring of vitamin B-12 status. Clin Chim Acta. 2002 Dec;326(1-2):47-59

[350] Pepper MR, Black MM. B12 in fetal development. Semin Cell Dev Biol. 2011 Aug;22(6):619-23

[351] Fusco D, Colloca G, Lo Monaco MR, Cesari M. Effects of antioxidant supplementation on the aging process. Clin Interv Aging. 2007;2(3):377-87

[352] Sohal RS, Allen RG. Oxidative stress as a causal factor in differentiation and aging: a unifying hypothesis. Exp Gerontol. 1990;25(6):499-522

[353] The Harvard School of Public Health. Nutrition insurance policy: a multivitamin-multimineral supplement can fill in micronutrient gaps in your diet, October, 2010: http://www.hsph.harvard.edu/nutritionsource

[354] Green GA. Understanding NSAIDs: from aspirin to COX-2. Clin Cornerstone. 2001;3(5):50-60

[355] Reginster JY, Deroisy R, Rovati LC, Lee RL, Lejeune E, Bruyere O, Giacovelli G, Henrotin Y, Dacre JE, Gossett C. Long-term effects of glucosamine sulphate on osteoarthritis progression: a randomised, placebo-controlled clinical trial. Lancet. 2001 Jan 27;357(9252):251-6

[356] Pavelká K, Gatterová J, Olejarová M, Machacek S, Giacovelli G, Rovati LC. Glucosamine sulfate use and delay of progression of knee osteoarthritis: a 3-year, randomized, placebo-controlled, double-blind study. Arch Intern Med. 2002 Oct 14;162(18):2113-23

[357] Clegg DO, Reda DJ, Harris CL, Klein MA, O'Dell JR, Hooper MM, Bradley JD, Bingham CO 3rd, Weisman MH, Jackson CG, Lane NE, Cush JJ, Moreland LW, Schumacher HR Jr, Oddis CV, Wolfe F, Molitor JA, Yocum DE, Schnitzer TJ, Furst DE, Sawitzke AD, Shi H, Brandt KD, Moskowitz RW, Williams HJ. Glucosamine, chondroitin sulfate, and the two in combination for painful knee osteoarthritis. N Engl J Med. 2006 Feb 23;354(8):795-808

[358] National Center for Complimentary and Alternative Medicine. The NIH Glucosamine/Chondroitin Arthritis Intervention Trial (GAIT). J Pain Palliat Care Pharmacother. 2008;22(1):39-43

[359] Bruyere O, Reginster JY. Glucosamine and chondroitin sulfate as therapeutic agents for knee and hip osteoarthritis. Drugs Aging. 2007;24(7):573-80

[360] Lee YH, Woo JH, Choi SJ, Ji JD, Song GG. Effect of glucosamine or chondroitin sulfate on the osteoarthritis progression: a meta-analysis. Rheumatol Int. 2010 Jan;30(3):357-63

361 Wandel S, Jüni P, Tendal B, Nüesch E, Villiger PM, Welton NJ, Reichenbach S, Trelle S. Effects of glucosamine, chondroitin, or placebo in patients with osteoarthritis of hip or knee: network meta-analysis. BMJ. 2010 Sep 16;341:c4675

362 Gregory PJ, Fellner C. Dietary supplements as disease-modifying treatments in osteoarthritis: a critical appraisal. P T. 2014 Jun;39(6):436-52

363 MacDougall JD. Morphological changes in human skeletal muscle following strength training and immobilization. *Human Muscle Strength*, Jones NL, McCartney N, McComas AJ, eds. Human Kinetics: Champaign, IL. 1986, pp. 269-288

364 Rawson ES, Volek JS. Effects of creatine supplementation and resistance training on muscle strength and weightlifting performance. J Strength Cond Res. 2003 Nov;17(4):822-31

365 Wyss M, Kaddurah-Daouk R. Creatine and creatinine metabolism. Physiol Rev. 2000 Jul;80(3):1107-213

366 Balsom PD, Söderlund K, Ekblom B. Creatine in humans with special reference to creatine supplementation. Sports Med. 1994 Oct;18(4):268-80

367 Selsby JT, DiSilvestro RA, Devor ST. Mg2+-creatine chelate and a low-dose creatine supplementation regimen improve exercise performance. J Strength Cond Res. 2004 May;18(2):311-5

368 Kendall KL, Smith AE, Graef JL, Fukuda DH, Moon JR, Beck TW, Cramer JT, Stout JR. Effects of four weeks of high-intensity interval training and creatine supplementation on critical power and anaerobic working capacity in college-aged men. J Strength Cond Res. 2009 Sep;23(6):1663-9

369 Cooper R, Naclerio F, Allgrove J, Jimenez A. Creatine supplementation with specific view to exercise/sports performance: an update. J Int Soc Sports Nutr. 2012 Jul 20;9(1):33

370 Hultman E, Söderlund K, Timmons JA, Cederblad G, Greenhaff PL. Muscle creatine loading in men. J Appl Physiol. 1996 Jul;81(1):232-7

371 LeBlanc J, Jobin M, Côté J, Samson P, Labrie A. Enhanced metabolic response to caffeine in exercise-trained human subjects. J Appl Physiol. 1985 Sep;59(3):832-7

372 Costill DL, Dalsky GP, Fink WJ. Effects of caffeine ingestion on metabolism and exercise performance. Med Sci Sports. 1978 Fall;10(3):155-8

373 Van Soeren MH, Sathasivam P, Spriet LL, Graham TE. Caffeine metabolism and epinephrine responses during exercise in users and nonusers. J Appl Physiol. 1993 Aug;75(2):805-12

374 Vandenberghe K, Gillis N, Van Leemputte M, Van Hecke P, Vanstapel F, Hespel P. Caffeine counteracts the ergogenic action of muscle creatine loading. J Appl Physiol. 1996 Feb;80(2):452-7

375 Crinnion WJ. Organic foods contain higher levels of certain nutrients, lower levels of pesticides, and may provide health benefits for the consumer. Altern Med Rev. 2010 Apr;15(1):4-12

376 Smith-Spangler C, Brandeau ML, Hunter GE, Bavinger JC, Pearson M, Eschbach PJ, Sundaram V, Liu H, Schirmer P, Stave C, Olkin I, Bravata DM. Are organic foods safer or healthier than conventional alternatives?: a systematic review. Ann Intern Med. 2012 Sep 4;157(5):348-66

377 Environmental Working Group. Shopper's guide to pesticides in produce: the dirty dozen. Environmental Working Group, 2012

378 Organic Gardening Magazine. Organic gardening holds water. Rodale Press, 400 South Tenth St., Emmaus PA 18098-0099. http://www.organicgardening.com/living/organic-methods-hold-water

379 Segasothy M, Phillips PA. Vegetarian diet: panacea for modern lifestyle diseases? QJM. 1999 Sep;92(9):531-44

380 Wyatt HR, Grunwald GK, Mosca CL, Klem ML, Wing RR, Hill JO. Long-term weight loss and breakfast in subjects in the National Weight Control Registry. Obes Res. 2002 Feb;10(2):78-82

381 López-Alt JK. So You Like Flavor? Don't Soak Your Black Beans! http://seriouseats.com/2014/09/soaking-black-beans-faq.html

382 Seal CJ, Brownlee IA. Whole-grain foods and chronic disease: evidence from epidemiological and intervention studies. Proc Nutr Soc. 2015 Aug;74(3):313-9

383 University of Missouri-Columbia News Bureau, Daily Dog Walks Work Off Weight for Owners, http://www.cvm.missouri.edu/News/dailydogwalks.htm

384 TV-Turnoff Network. Facts and figures about our TV habit. TV-Turnoff Network, 1200 29th St NW, LL #1, Washington DC 20007. http://tvturnoff.org/images/facts&figs/factsheets/FactsFigs.pdf

385 Robinson TN. Reducing children's television viewing to prevent obesity: a randomized controlled trial. JAMA. 1999 Oct 27;282(16):1561-7